Discover the New You

Discover the New You

Celebrity stylist secrets
to transform your life and style

Ceril Campbell

bookshaker

First Published In Great Britain 2011
by www.BookShaker.com

© Copyright Ceril Campbell
Illustrations by Christopher Page

This book is dedicated to Arabella and Rory, my two wonderful children, and my favourite Auntie Sylvia, who have all always been there for me as I have tried to be for them.

For attractive lips,

Speak words of kindness.

For lovely eyes,

Seek out the good in people.

For a slim figure,

Share your food with the hungry.

For beautiful hair,

Let a child run his/her fingers through it once a day.

For poise,

Walk with the knowledge that you never walk alone.

People, even more than things,

Have to be restored, renewed, revived, reclaimed,

And redeemed; never throw out anyone.

Remember, if you ever need a helping hand,

You will find one at the end of each of your arms.

As you grow older, you will discover that you have two hands;

One for helping yourself, and the other for helping others.

Audrey Hepburn

People, even more than things, have to be restored, renewed, revived, reclaimed, and redeemed; never throw out anyone " – I love this quote from Audrey Hepburn; it epitomises everything I believe in and have written about in this book. Beauty comes from within. If you feel happy, confident and positive, others will perceive you as a beautiful person. That is far more important that being only a beautiful face.

Ceril Campbell

Contents

* * * * * * * * * * *

Introduction

You would like to discover a new you. But how can you do it?

When you aren't happy with yourself and your life, but don't know how to change your circumstances, who can you talk to? Friends and family are often not those you wish to take advice from. You either won't listen to them, they won't listen to you, or they are too close to the problem. How do you find someone who can look deeper within you and strike a chord that you can relate to?

Maybe you don't want a dramatic change; just a tweak to your life, in the same way you might go to a spa to pamper yourself and give yourself a 'spring clean' or detox.

Wanting to change how you feel about yourself and how others perceive you can happen any time, whatever your age. This realisation could be a seed of thought that has gradually been growing over months or years, fuelled by a lack of self-esteem, weight gain or loss or an unhappy relationship. It could also be brought on by a sudden shock caused by betrayal, divorce, job redundancy, bereavement, illness, reaching a birthday milestone or empty nest syndrome.

With the ever increasing pace of life, the instant fix is the easy option. Whether you choose the latest lunch hour plastic surgery that promises you a more youthful look, or internet dating to find that elusive soul mate, neither solves the longer term issue of personal life change. To be happy and self-fulfilled you need to discover *yourself* first.

So how can you discover yourself?

I can help you and work with you in the same way as I have worked with my celebrity clients. You can discover who *you* really are, both your inner and outer you. You can find out how you see yourself and how others see you; how you can make small changes that may be invisible to others but that can make a big difference to you.

I will ask you, as I have done with my celebrity clients, a series of questions. My solutions for your 'best you' are based on your responses. So you will need to select responses that you most identify with and you will find your personal solution.

In this way you can continue your journey to 'discovering the new you' as though I am actually with you, holding your hand all the way.

This is not a quick fix book, but one where you will be taking a step-by-step journey with me, where the final destination is your best you. On the way, you will be evaluating yourself and at various crossroads choosing the direction you want to take. This book is the vehicle for your journey of discovery with me. My aim is that when you have finished the book, you can continue on your journey with the confidence that you deserve.

I have written this book drawing on my 30 years of experience with my celebrity and personal image and lifestyle clients. I have listened, watched and taken on board my clients' feelings about their body shape issues, self-doubts, lack of self-esteem, confidence, relationships and all the facets of how they feel about themselves and how others see them. You don't have to be perfect to make the most of yourself. As Elizabeth Arden said, 'Every woman deserves to be beautiful'.

My work has given me an insight into the psychology of feeling as good within yourself and as you may appear to others. In my capacity as a celebrity stylist and image consultant, the most amazing doors have been opened for me, giving me a chance not only to discover the beauty and style secrets of A list stars, but also to work with them to hide their imperfections and insecurities.

I have met and worked with some of the most famous and glamorous people in the world, from sports stars to movie stars to royalty. Celebrities that I have styled over 30 years for Red Carpet appearances, TV and photo shoots include Jane Seymour, Ringo Starr, Darcey Bussell CBE, Richard Branson, Anna Kournikova, Dannii Minogue, Katherine Jenkins and Princess Anne's daughter, Zara Phillips (you can visit my website, www.cerilcampbell.com, to see more of the celebrities I have worked with).

I have been backstage at fashion shows and theatres; inside royal palaces; stayed in desert locations and five star hotels; walked down the red carpet and partied with stars; and been allowed to rummage inside celebrities' closets. My favourite closet was Ringo Starr's and his Beatles' vintage clothes.

I was never intimidated or overawed to work with big name celebrities. When you work with stars you realise that they are only human and have the same lack of self-esteem and feelings about their bodies as all of us. In fact they are even more insecure as they're faced with the media picking apart their appearance. The public image of the celebrities you see is not how they look on a daily basis. This perfection is created with the help of airbrushing in photos and a team of stylists, hair and makeup artists. This is not real life. Even the celebrities often don't recognise themselves in their airbrushed pictures!

Whether you're male or female, celebrity or not, looking good is not simply about being fit, stylish or wearing the latest designer label, but about attitude, confidence, and feeling good within.

You don't have to be the best looking person in the room to attract or make people interested in you. But if you believe in yourself and feel good, you will exude an inner confidence and most importantly the magnetic power of attraction. This attraction is not about drawing people to you in a sexual way, but giving off a magnetic aura. If you are able to make people think that you are the most interesting person in the room, then you will be able to make new friends and business contacts for the future.

You can't expect to gain confidence and become a new person overnight, or even in a month, but you can improve on who you are in gradual steps.

Don't get overwhelmed by these steps to the new you. Once you feel good about yourself, anything is possible. Set yourself your new standards and small goals in baby steps, especially if you feel that you lost yourself somewhere along the way. Your goal could be, 'I will lose a few pounds by the end of this month' or 'I will give myself an hour a day especially for me'. This hour could be to do anything, even just sitting doing absolutely nothing if you are constantly stressed and frantic during the rest of the day. This book is not about me preaching to you, but understanding the issues that we all have and taking the journey together with you. I have learnt a lot from my own life's ups and downs, (and there have been many over the years – including divorce, after a 20-year marriage, the death of both aged parents, moving home five times in three years and various health problems with both my children), so I hope that I am able to impart to you what my life experiences and, of course, those of my clients have taught me.

As soon as you start to invest in yourself, everything in your life will start to fall into place. If you water and nurture seedlings, they put down strong roots and become beautiful plants. In the same way, if you look after yourself, you can become the 'new you'.

Ceril Campbell

Part One

The Inner You

. . . .

**How you feel about yourself
and how others perceive you**

The first stage of the journey to the new you

Make the most of yourself, for that is all there is of you.
Ralph Waldo Emerson

*He who knows others is clever. He who knows himself is
enlightened.* Lao Tzu

*Everyone thinks of changing the world but no one thinks
of changing himself.* Leo Tolstoy

*I can change. I can live my imagination instead of my
memory. I can tie myself to my limitless potential
instead of my limiting past.'* Stephen Covey

On the first stage of your journey with me, I want you to find out how you *feel* about yourself. How you *see* yourself and how you think others see you. Do you just feel that you've lost your sense of style and you don't know how to dress for your age or for a changing body shape?

Or does your problem run deeper? How do you feel about the inner you and the outer physical you? How do you feel about your personal relationships and your relationships with food, alcohol, shopping, exercise and even sex?

Do you always say to yourself that you are going to start that diet, give up smoking, or begin the exercise regime tomorrow – never today? Do you always have excuses for yourself, or have these daily activities become addictions that create an adrenalin rush or a feeling of instant gratification?

Have you always had low or no self-esteem or how and when did it disappear? Do you look in the mirror and say to yourself, 'I'm not worth it'?

You could find you have a completely distorted view of your self-image. I have styled many celebrities and 'real' women who are beautiful and successful, but still have no self-confidence.

> *I have exactly the same issues and hang-ups as any woman would have going down the red carpet. You know, what if I step on my train and tear my dress? What if I get my period? That's why a backup black dress is essential. When I read how an actress "made a statement in black", I just think, "Oh, period or fat day".*

Sometimes you just don't feel confident enough to wear twinkly yellow taffeta.

Kate Winslet

How can you define what is wrong with both you and your life that you'd like to change? How can you step outside your life and look in?

Try making lists with category headings. The first heading and column should include all those things that you like about yourself and your life. All those positive things you wouldn't want to change. Even if you can't find very many, there must be some. The second column should include those things that you are able to change that can make an instant difference. The third column should have all the things that you can change over time. Writing down your wishes and needs can often help clarify your thoughts.

Positive things that you like about your life that you don't want to change	Things you can change that would make an instant difference	Things you could change over time
your children your family good eyes your sense of humour good boobs	de-clutter your life (e.g. rooms in the home, personal belongings, 'friends' in your address book) get a new haircut/colour	look for a new job move house, move town improve your body shape with exercise and a healthy, nutritional diet

	buy good underwear that makes you feel sexy	work on your current relationship with your partner or husband
	put five minutes a day aside for 'you' time	find a new lover/partner/relationship
	get contact lenses instead of glasses	
	go out more	
	find someone to babysit the children one night a week	
	have a weekly 'date' night with your long term partner	

> *Ask the right questions if you're to find the right answers.*
>
> Vanessa Redgrave

You can't wait for someone else to rescue you, or a life-changing solution to suddenly appear out of the blue. You are responsible for your own life and you create your own destiny. If you want change in any area of your life, you are the only one who can make it happen.

It's a bit like an overgrown garden full of weeds. If you clear the weeds away, creating space and light for new plant shoots, they will have a chance to grow. With no light or space, they will be suffocated and die. If you create the space in your life for new opportunities and possibilities for change, then these changes can have a chance to happen. In the same way, de-cluttering your home could give it a whole new feel – maybe one that is more suited to your new life as the 'new you'.

If you confide in a close friend or someone you trust to share your thoughts and feelings, you may often find that you are not alone in those negative thoughts of how you feel about your body/your life/your partner or even your mortality. When you realise that there are others who feel the same, sometimes it helps you rationalise your thoughts. A negative head, or 'poor me' syndrome will drag you down. Optimism will help you look ahead and see exciting new and positive things (however small) that happen to you each day, and you can build on them. To help create positivity, you could try writing down 10 reasons that make *you* unique.

> *Life is about creating new opportunities,*
> *not waiting for them to come to you.*
>
> Salma Hayek

Be patient. It takes lots of little steps to make a long journey, in the same way as a day in your life is made up of lots of little details and events.

How do you see yourself?

I'm worthless.
Have you let yourself go because you feel that you are worthless? Have you stopped taking any exercise and caring

for your body, telling yourself, 'Why should anyone else be interested in me if I'm worthless?'

Have you immersed yourself in caring for your children/your aged or infirm parents to the exclusion of everything else? Have you forgotten about *you*?

How can you escape from this vicious circle? You are unhappy, you turn to food or alcohol. The more you eat the fatter you become. You look in the mirror and can't bear to look at yourself, then become unhappier and repeat the cycle.

How can you break a pattern which may have been continuing for years? Has it gone on for so long that you can't see how to change it?

Or have you tried and failed already? Maybe you've given yourself too great a task. Maybe you expect a change in too short a time. If a problem has been continuing on for years then you can't fix it in a day, a week or even a month. It needs to become a long-term plan taken in little steps. The equivalent of a great football goal, achieved with lots of little passes to get close enough to score safely.

I don't like myself.
Do you look in the mirror and hate what you see? What is it that you dislike? Is it your boobs, your tummy, or maybe your bum? Do you think you are too thin, too fat, disproportionate, too tall, too short? According to statistics, 50 per cent of you have low self-esteem and judge yourselves harshly, even if no one else is being critical of you.

Seeing and liking yourself is not about seeing your actual reflection in the mirror, but about how you perceive the whole of you from your personality to your body shape.

You need to accept the physical you. It's all about your mental attitude. If you think more positively, then you will find that it's easier to move on with your life with renewed confidence. I want you to look in the mirror and love what you see.

> *If everybody's not a beauty,*
> *then nobody is.*
>
> Andy Warhol

I'm uninteresting, unattractive, useless and unlovable.
Why don't you *like* you? Do you have a little voice repeatedly telling you that you're uninteresting, unattractive, useless, maybe even unlovable? Were these thoughts planted in your head by a partner, a family member or your school classmates from years ago? These thought patterns may have been reinforced with repetition over the years, gradually eroding your self-esteem.

How can you start to believe the positive and get rid of the negative? You'll need to see yourself in a positive light to be able to turn things around and after years of negativity it can take a while to become positive again.

My husband or partner ignored me so I ignored
my own needs.
You must always feel good and look good for *you*, not anyone else. But if you are constantly rejected, criticised or ignored

it will be very difficult to regain confidence and step out of that cycle. But with the knowledge that only you can help yourself, then it is important to remember that you owe it to yourself to tend to yourself and your needs, as you would weed and make over a neglected and overgrown garden. It might take time for the flowers to grow again and the lawn to look healthy and green- but it will do, in the same way that you can look good again.

> *If I hadn't been a fat teenager, I would never have been funny. If I had been as skinny as one of those supermodels I would never have developed my sense of humour.*
>
> Joan Rivers

I hate my body!
Do you really have a body image that you dislike enough to never undress in front of anyone, even your girlfriends or husband? Do you always undress in another room or in the dark? What is it that you don't like? Have you discussed it with your husband/partner/girlfriends? Would it be true to say that they all tell you that you look OK and your husband/partner keeps telling you how much he loves you and all the bits of you for who you are, but you still don't listen...?

The more you focus on those few parts of your body you do like and really listen to the positive reinforcement and compliments from your partner and friends, you may suddenly see the body that others see, not the one you conjure up in your mind. Others only see you as a whole and how you present yourself and project your personality.

I don't believe my friends and family when they say nice things about me.
Listen to your friends and family when they compliment you and accept it. If someone says how pretty you look, feel it! If you're praised for something you did, then realise that it *was* good. If someone writes you a letter complimenting you on something you did, keep it to read every time you feel lacking in self-confidence. They meant what they wrote in the letter. I have a simple, fun group exercise in my Discover the New You workshops that helps everyone see how others perceive them. Everyone always leaves my workshops with a smile on their face from reinforced positivity.

I compare myself to others.
Challenge or compete with yourself but don't compare yourself to others. You would be surprised what others may feel about themselves, however pretty or successful they may be. Most of the advertising images that your see daily, showing perfect women, have been digitally enhanced. Therefore, if you compare yourself to them, you will become more critical of yourself, with an unreasonable image and perception of how you feel you should look.

> *Even I don't look like Claudia Schiffer.*
> Claudia Schiffer

But how many perfect women have you seen in reality? Maybe models in magazines and women under the age of 25, but I can guarantee that although you may perceive them as perfect, they too will be obsessing with at least one area of their bodies.

Every person whom I have ever styled, even the most glamorous Hollywood actresses you see on the red carpet, has body shape issues. So let's look at the positive. What do you like most about yourself when you look in the mirror? Be realistic. You don't have to be perfect. The imperfections of the actresses and personalities you see on magazine pages have all been airbrushed out.

There must be something you can find to like about yourself... Your décolleté? How about your shoulders or your ankles? Focus on that area and make those who look at you do the same.

> *When you know people are going to see all your blobby bits in the press, it makes it all worse. Some days you wake up feeling thin and pretty, other days you feel awful. I've got wobbly bits that I hate and I'm as embarrassed by my figure as any woman. I never feel gorgeous.*

Joss Stone

There is huge pressure for both women and men to look a certain way and use beauty products. You are supposed to be ultra thin, successful and look eternally youthful. You should aspire to the latest fashion trend, 'must have' handbag or Jimmy Choo shoe. Young girls are targeted by magazines to use the latest make-up, whilst women are being told to consider cosmetic surgery even when they are in their twenties.

> *I refuse to become part of this perfect body syndrome. I like my body. It looks good on-screen, and it's not because it's perfect. I accept it and wear it like a good dress... One guy I dated said: "You're beautiful but you're soft. You can't compete with other actresses in Hollywood because everyone's in shape and working out." I said: "Very nice to meet you. Goodbye!"*
>
> Salma Hayek

We all want what we haven't got. We would like straight hair instead of curly, a big bust instead of small, and to be beautiful. But the grass isn't always greener. Many beautiful women feel cursed by their beauty, not blessed.

> *The director may tell me it looks perfect, but I always find that stray hair or eyebrow. I can't wait for my looks to fade.*
>
> Jennifer Lopez

> *I cried myself to sleep wishing I was ugly because men leered and disrespected me.*
>
> Evangeline Lily of Lost

> *People are frightened by beautiful people. My friends never want to meet me in my office because they are scared of the models. Beauty creates an immediate barrier, but the reality is that behind it is a perfectly normal person. It's a wonderful thing that we all look different.*
>
> Sarah Doukas, Storm modelling agency

It's not easy to be beautiful, as often the most beautiful people are the most self-conscious, and always being stared at. Their looks may be their trademark, their life, their career. And as they age, they have to deal with losing their best asset.

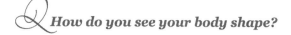

How do you see your body shape?

I worry about my body shape.

If you do, you are not alone. We seem to have reached a point where the word 'fat' is taboo and we are immune to true beauty, which can appear in all shapes and sizes.

> *It feels like I have somehow fooled everybody and managed to cover up the misshapen strange child for an evening.*
>
> Kate Beckinsale

Do you know what your body shape is, or do you simply know that you don't like it?

But which part of your body is it that you don't like? Your boobs, your bum, the cellulite on your thighs or your actual body shape structure? Or do you feel that it's just all one big problem?

Your basic body shape is your skeletal make-up. You can change how thin or fat you are, but you cannot change your bone structure. You're stuck with it. But you can improve your body shape 'casing' by slimming, toning, dealing with cellulite and looking after your skin. So put aside any thoughts of those bits you dislike and look again.

In Part Two, we will find out your body shape. Once you have established your shape, you can work on making the best of it with styling, cut and colour of your clothes. Dressing cleverly can create an illusion of a different body shape. Knowing which shape you are can help you to look your best.

I can't bear to look in the mirror.

Do you hate what you have become so much that you never look in the mirror? Or even at yourself when you're in the bath? Your body may not be what it used to be, but there is no reason why you can't improve it with exercise, good eating habits and body care. Yes, stretch marks may happen with pregnancy and everything gradually going south comes with age, but life is for living. Just consider how empty your life would be without your wonderful kids and how much pleasure they give you. Just because your body isn't perfect doesn't mean than you can't still be attractive, even beautiful. Beauty is not just superficial.

> *Someone with the perfect body may just be a bunch of perfect parts.*
>
> Matthew Mcconaughey

When you look in the mirror, are you truthful to yourself and do you really see what you're looking at, or are you in denial? Do you see yourself as the size 10 woman you once were, when you're really now a size 16? Or do you see yourself as an overweight woman, when it's simply your tummy that carries the pounds and the rest of you is tall and slim?

Obviously you can't change your height or your bone structure but you can change how you perceive yourself. You may find that the reality could be better than the 'imagined you'. Many of my clients who have achieved a significant weight loss still think of themselves as a few sizes bigger. They are really shocked when I select clothes the correct size which happen to be a few sizes less than they think they are.

However slim you become, do you still see yourself as fat? Do you look at your body and actually hate it? Do you never undress in front of anyone, your family, your friends or your husband or partner? Is sex always with the lights off? How can you overcome this problem which is all in your mind, especially if your body shape in other people's eyes is quite OK?

Body dysmorphic disorder

Seeing yourself in the mirror not as your true size but as your imagined size (which to you may seem non-negotiable, however much anyone tries to convince you otherwise) is a form of body dysmorphic disorder.

If you are anorexic, you may only see a fat person in the mirror, even if you only weigh seven stone. Equally, if you have low self-esteem you may imagine your body to be unattractive, when in reality it is perfectly acceptable.

It may be almost as if you are two different people. One is maybe the self you recognise from way back and the other is the self you find shocking to see in the mirror, as it is not the 'ideal' you have in your mind. To like yourself more you have to accept that some flesh/fat is essential. Wanting to be a better person is a positive thing, but wanting to be thinner will not make you a better person.

Most people with body dysmorphic disorder also have eating disorders, such as bulimia or anorexia. It may be that these psychological issues need to be resolved before you see yourself how others see you, so that you can see your true reflection in the mirror, not a distorted one.

I am having a 'feeling fat' day.
A 'fat' *day* is not about how you look but about how you feel. No one else would actually see any difference in your body, but you could feel like a beached whale. Of course all women have times of the month when the body changes due to menstrual cycles, and maybe you do get water retention and carry an extra few pounds that week, but this is not a 'feeling fat' day. A 'feeling fat' day is triggered by your insecurity, your

lack of confidence and low sense of worth. Maybe you might be lonely, bored or dissatisfied. A 'feeling fat' day can also be brought on by stress or a negative comment.

On these days you will imagine you see parts of your body as disproportionately large and think that everyone else is focussing on these parts too. Whether you target your tummy or your thighs as your fat parts, you'll decide to wear baggy or black clothes to cover them up and do extra exercise that day. These areas will become everything that you hate about yourself.

How can I stop having a feeling fat day?
Be aware that wearing baggy clothes, weighing yourself and checking yourself constantly in the mirror will make you feel worse. Be less judgemental and look at the things that you like about yourself that you know haven't changed from the preceding day, such as your eyes, your hair colour, your skin etc.

Stop imagining that everyone is only looking at your 'fat' bottom, thighs or your tummy. Could there be another reason they are looking? Maybe you are attractive or even glamorous, but don't realise it. Maybe you have a large bust which you hate, but others would love to have, or fantastic hair?

Try and remember and consider all your positive personal attributes and qualities and base your self-worth on those rather than your appearance. It will raise your self-esteem and confidence and those 'feeling fat' days may eventually disappear or become less stressful and more manageable.

Can I change my shape with better posture?

With incorrect posture, you can reveal to others how you feel about yourself. If you have low self-esteem, it is very likely that you don't hold yourself proudly. Do you slump in your seat? Do you stand with your torso concertinaed into your hips, making your bust droop and tummy sick out? Or do you stand in an 'S' shape, with tummy and bum out and a sway back? Good posture can create a better body shape, lose pounds instantly and also make your body look better proportioned. If you stand up proud and pull up from your waist, you will look more confident and have more of a presence in a room. In my Discover the New You group workshops I teach how to stand and pose for the camera- and then show the before and after pictures. My ladies can never believe the difference good posture makes.

If you are lacking in confidence from how you may have been treated by a super-critical ex-partner, it will be even more important for you to really look at yourself in the mirror and focus on the positive. No one is perfect.

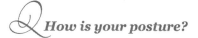

How is your posture?

I hate my large bust and try to hide it by how I stand.

Even if you are self-conscious, shy or hate some part of your body don't try to hide it with your arms or your stance. If you hate your large bust, don't stand slouched to try and hide it. You won't, you will only give yourself a droopy bust and

23

sloping shoulders. Properly fitted lingerie will make all the difference to your posture, comfort and even body shape under your clothes.

I slouch as I think I am too tall.
If you are tall, don't try to hide your height by standing slouched. Tall girls rarely stand tall as they were teased at school, so they carry on trying to look shorter. The shy young Princess Diana was an example of a young woman who began her public life with bad stance as she felt tall and also had a big bust. As she became more confident her posture improved and she walked and stood tall, looking glamorous and confident, even if she wasn't feeling confident inside. Nicole Kidman commented after her split from Tom Cruise, that finally she could wear heels again as she had previously been too concerned about being taller than her man.

I try to hide my tummy.
If you feel your tummy is too large, don't sit with your arms crossed to hide it when you're seated. Try sitting up more and pulling in instead. It will help remind your tummy muscles to get working again. If you have a short-waisted body shape, the more you stand up, the more it will lengthen the space between your chest and tummy. It will also lengthen a shorter neck, lift your bust (without surgery) and give you back a waist.

I lack confidence so maybe I subconsciously slouch.

Do you slouch and try to pretend you're invisible? Stand up straight, shoulders back, with hips, knees and arms loose and eyes ahead. If you look relaxed and comfortable in your own skin, you will appear more confident and attractive.

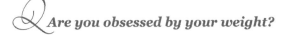

Are you obsessed by your weight?

I feel really fat.

Have you noticed a gradual weight gain that you felt you couldn't control? Do you have long-term unworn clothes hanging in your wardrobe, as they are for the other, thinner you? Maybe you do carry a few excess pounds, have boobs that have drooped, or a tummy that bears the tale of your pregnancies. But don't imagine that your current partner or future partner will focus on this area when they look at you; they won't. They will simply see the whole you and like or love you unconditionally for who you are. The most beautiful celebrities have insecurities about all sorts of parts of their body, even body parts that most of you wouldn't begin to consider a problem!

> *I don't like my hands because my knuckles are too big.*
> *If I get married, I'm worried that the ring won't fit.*
> Eva Longoria

However much exercise I do I can't shift those last few pounds.

You should never weigh yourself every day as your weight will fluctuate according to the time of the month and what you ate the preceding day, and even if you've been to the loo! Muscle weighs more than fat and if you have been losing fat by exercise you will have been gaining muscle instead. You should look at yourself in the mirror undressed and then try on your clothes. How they fit will tell you how your weight loss is progressing. You may find that you actually don't need to lose those extra pounds; you are absolutely fine as you are. There are many celebrities who are in denial about their weight. Try to see you as you really are. If you think you may have an eating disorder, it is important to seek help.

Have you ever asked yourself why you're eating, when you're not actually hungry? Is snacking your only treat? Is eating the only time you let yourself be out of control? Does eating fire up your senses and become a sensual or gratifying experience? When you do give into your cravings and needs, do you feel the need to binge? If you have an addictive personality, when you give up something it's likely that you will find an alternative addiction. So you need to find a balance.

It's all about being less hard on yourself and allowing yourself a small amount of those things you crave within reason, without completely cutting them out. It shouldn't be an all or nothing scenario. That's why diets never work. You should be able to enjoy a small bar of chocolate once a week or an occasional glass of wine without beating yourself up.

So how do you change your mindset about food so that *you* use *it*, instead of *it* using *you*?

> *Everyone would talk about their diets, and what it made me do was go and eat. I immediately went to the drugstore and bought a bunch of cookies. I wanted to rebel.*
>
> Kristin Davis talks about her *Sex and the City* days.

> *One of the best exercises for losing weight is the "push-yourself-away-from-the-dining-room-table-before-you-eat-too-much" exercise.*
>
> Joan Collins

How is your relationship with food?

Is food your friend? But what sort of friend? One you turn to when you're depressed or stressed or lonely? Or is it more of an addictive or abusive relationship? You should know when to walk away from any abusive relationship and get help. In the same way, you should be able to enjoy your food and walk away, still leaving some on your plate.

Everyone is human and everyone has imperfections and emotional vulnerability. So why try to be perfect? Be kinder and more forgiving on yourself and you may find that you don't need to seek the comfort of the food, alcohol or drugs or even shopping that you may use to dull your emotions..

I eat when I'm unhappy, stressed or just bored.

You need to be aware what triggers your desire to eat when it's not hunger driven, and find something that occupies that moment instead. You probably need to make sure that you are as far away from the kitchen or food temptation as possible. Try going out for a short brisk walk (as exercise helps produce the endorphins or happy feelings). Or even have a chat on the phone with a friend. Anything that helps distract you from the instant gratification that eating will give you.

> *What's the difference between single women and married women? Single women go home, see what's in the fridge and then go to bed. Married women go home, see what's in the bed and then go to the fridge.*
>
> Unknown

I think if I eat I will put on all my weight again.

You need to understand why and when you eat. Always have breakfast. It sets you up for the day. If you need a mid-morning snack and you really know you aren't able to control your urge for only one biscuit, don't have any at all and substitute an alternative, healthier nibbling choice. Always try to exercise before you eat a meal as the exercise will raise your metabolism. When you eat you will burn up the calories quicker.

Shaping up, starting to exercise

How do you get in the mindset to start exercise? Once you start and create some semblance of a routine, even if its only 20 minutes a few times a week, you will find that the action of exercise triggers endorphins and you will start to feel good about yourself after the exercising. As the weeks pass, you will see changes in your body which will make you feel even better about yourself. Looking good is all about feeling good which comes from within. So in the end, it doesn't really matter what size you are as long as you feel good about how you look. It's unlikely that you need to be as toned as Madonna, who apparently does do three hours working out a day. You only need to be fit enough to have a flatter tum, a perkier bum and eliminate those under-arm bingo wings.

See Part Two for more about starting to exercise.

Do you feel depressed?

I feel depressed as I have no confidence or self-esteem.
If you lack self-esteem, however many times your friends tell you that you're pretty, you still aren't going to believe them. You will still see yourself as that unattractive person in your mind. Maybe you had a prettier, cleverer, older sister, or a more handsome, higher achieving, brother, or parents who had a higher expectation of you than you felt you could ever achieve. Or conversely parents who didn't care.

So how can you increase your confidence? How can you see

what others see in you? Try not to compete with anyone other than yourself and each time you succeed in something, give yourself a mental point as a reward. This success could be anything from finally getting into that pair of jeans you bought that were too tight, attracting someone you've been fancying for ages, to jogging for an extra 10 minutes longer than usual. You will soon find those points keep clocking up, and the sense of achievement will boost your inner confidence.

Being at home depresses me.
If you can't get out of the house, you will feel more depressed as you will feel caged in. Even a five minute breath of fresh air and quick walk, even just round the block, will help renew your energy. Some sort of exercise will help elevate your mood. Being in and seeing sunlight/daylight will help, especially if you live in a dark home.

Is your home too small? Maybe de-cluttering would help, as it will make the rooms seem bigger. Redecorating a dark, dingy room to be a light, bright one will give it a much happier feel.

If certain rooms do lower your spirits, it could be the colour of them that is affecting how you feel. Certain colours will be more uplifting. Yellow creates a sunshine-happy feel, whilst red creates energy. Blues and greens and lilacs are tranquil and calming. A bedroom should always be a calming and tranquil-coloured environment, helping you to sleep peacefully.

Self-esteem

How do you feel about yourself? Do you have self-esteem? Do you like who you are or do you feel that you are worthless and unattractive? Self-esteem is the most important thing that you can have. With self-esteem it doesn't matter what anyone else says or does to you as you are secure in the knowledge that actually you are OK. It isn't about how you look or how successful you are, but just about the value you put on yourself.

When you value yourself, you have the confidence to be yourself, not to be a victim, to stand up to your bullies and to take control of your life and empower yourself.

I am stuck in a hopeless rut.
When you feel that you are stuck in a rut, how can you escape? Is the problem how you think you look, how you interact with people, or that you feel that your life is going nowhere?

So, what's your goal? Could you make a plan of action and achieve it? It doesn't have to be instantly attainable but should be something that could gradually happen over time, with little baby steps.

How about making another table? It could cover the various aspects of your life that need a change, i.e. home, family life, work, clothes, body and exercise, social life, love life. Under each heading you could then put all the things that you would like to change over time.

Home	Family life	Social life		
Tidy bedroom and wardrobes (not a difficult task – just something that maybe you keep putting off)	Husband or friend/ relation to do school run once a week to give you a break	Go and learn a new skill whilst making new friends.		

This list could contain anything, however small – even if it seems stupid, it may make a big change to YOU.

" *Men do not stumble over mountains,*
but over mole hills. "

Confucius

So how can you meet more people who can become new friends, or present yourself in a different way?

You should start to make the most of your contacts. Learn to network. Take care with how you dress and that all-important first impression you give to others. You don't need to be the smartest or most talented person in the room to get ahead, but if you sound confident enough, people will listen to you and believe in you.

It's important to always be optimistic and never lose hope. You need to be a glass half full person, not half empty. There is always tomorrow to pick yourself up and start again if today wasn't good.

Q *Is your lack of self-esteem connected to your personal relationships?*

I use sex to gain self-esteem.

Do you sleep with a man to make yourself feel desirable? It may make you feel wanted at the time, but it's the same as eating a large bar of chocolate. It only felt good while it lasted. A quick fix and then you felt empty again. You don't need a man to boost your confidence and prove to yourself that you are desirable and not a worthless human being. That knowledge of self-worth can only come from your inner you. You can't look to others as your prop.

Mental bullying has erased my self-esteem.

Are you being bullied? Do you forgive the bully (because you love them) each time they apologise? Do you only see their good points while all the time your self-esteem is being eroded?

It's common to lack self-esteem after being bullied as a child at school, as an adult in your workplace or in your own home by your partner. Bullies always pick on the vulnerable, as they know that they will not be challenged. Many bullies are those who are the weakest and pick on others to make themselves feel better. Mental bullying can often be subliminal and you may not realise that it is even happening at the time. It could be that your partner always undermines you. He or she may never reciprocate any loving or tenderness or, worse still, refuse or rebuff your sexual approaches. Any of these things will gradually erode your self-esteem, however strong it may have been in the beginning. Everyone needs some sort of confirmation of approval. It could be from your parents or your partner but repeated negativity will breed lack of self-esteem.

It's very difficult to ignore repeated criticism, especially if it is always negative. But if you can be aware of it, without taking it to heart, then you can decide over a period of time what you wish to do to address the problem. Do you have the confidence or means to walk away or escape from the person or situation? Or do you stay? A verbally abusive relationship can be as destructive as a physically abusive one.

I no longer have sex, as he doesn't seem to fancy me any more. Have you been with your partner for what seems an eternity and does sex no longer seem to be on the agenda? Does your partner tell you he no longer finds you attractive, or has fallen out of love with you? If you no longer have sex you may find that you argue more often, are likely to be more irritable and depressed and will start to lose your self-esteem.

Regular sex within a loving relationship, even if it's a quickie, can help a relationship stay the course. It can help you communicate, show affection and be energised. Everyone needs some bodily contact, even if it's only a hug.

When you have a problem in a relationship, it is very easy to get stuck in a cycle of blame and shame. Have you considered that you could also be responsible for the problems? Try to look at the problems from the outside.

Michael Douglas' recipe for a happy marriage:
Don't take it for granted – that's really important. It's all about mutual respect.

Forgiveness has to be a long term strategy. It's easy to become the weaker half of the story and once trapped in that, you can only go down, blinded by your own lack of self-worth.

Patti Boyd

Do you blame yourself or your partner? Perhaps you may be partly to blame; maybe you didn't pay enough attention to him because of your children or work pressures. It takes two to make a marriage or partnership work. The more you put into a marriage, the more you get back. Have you lost who you were along the way and are no longer a lover and friend to your partner?

> *I believe that everyone is the keeper of a dream – and by tuning into one another's secret hopes, we can become better friends, better partners, better parents, and better lovers.*
>
> Oprah Winfrey

I want to encourage you to remember who you once were, and who you can be again. If you can remember *who* you are, you will be better equipped to regain a loving relationship.

How do you think others see you?

> *Deep down I'm pretty superficial.*
>
> Ava Gardener

I don't know.

Have you ever considered how others see you? Do you think you see yourself in the same way as they do or would you be upset if they told you their view? When told how they see you, would you withdraw into yourself, or be shocked and try to change accordingly? Do you take criticism personally or is it water off the proverbial duck's back? So who can you ask the questions 'How do I appear to you? What did you think of me when you first met me?' Who can you trust to give you the truth, or at least an unbiased opinion? If you have close, platonic friends of the opposite sex, try them first. You may be pleasantly surprised to hear what positive things friends of the opposite sex have to say about you. You may get a more generous reply from a man than one of your female friends.

There is often an underlying element of competition from your same sex friends... call it survival of the fittest. You could be amazed at how even your best friends may be jealous of some aspects of your life, and therefore be more economical with the truth. But make it clear when you ask that you want the truth, nothing less. However good or bad the feedback is, it can only be positive, as you then have knowledge about yourself to work with.

I don't think they notice me.

Why don't you think you are noticed? Do you choose to dress in colours and styles to be invisible and to purposely fade into the background, or do you feel that you don't have the personality or looks to be noticed?

Or did your mother constantly criticise you and tell you, as you were growing up, that you weren't good looking, that you should lose weight or drop hints about your skin?

You need to believe in what you now see in the mirror and not listen to those old voices in your head. If you were that scrawny be-spectacled gangly teenager, or the one with the acne-covered face you couldn't hide, or the fat girl in the class... Look again. That's not who you now see in that mirror. Don't let that image be reflected back at you. Others were ugly ducklings too – it's up to you to see yourself as a beautiful swan.

It is important to be noticed. You may not want to be noticed in an obvious way, but you don't want to be ignored.

You need to be noticed to leave a positive impression. First impressions are important in this fast paced life we live, so it's vital that you present the 'best you' possible. The first impression that you give may influence a prospective employer, a new hot date or just making new friends.

I don't want to be noticed.

Are you so shy that you can't bear to draw attention to yourself? Are you worried that everyone is judging your every move, what you wear and what you say? If so, how can you overcome this state of mind?

Firstly you have to realise that many people are actually far more interested in themselves than others, and will be looking out for themselves as a result. So it's very likely that they won't have noticed that you blushed when introducing yourself, as their attention may have moved on already.

Are they judging what you wear? Possibly, because first impressions count... but turn it around in your mind... do *they* look that great? They may well be as shy as you but just hiding it better. It's always good to see things from the point of view of others. It helps you feel better about yourself.

Are you terrified of meeting someone because they are important? Remember that everyone is the same underneath, however famous. Try imagining them on the loo – it will help divert you from your shyness issues! Most celebrities I have worked with like being treated as normally as possible, and appreciate it when you don't tiptoe around them with compliments and sycophancy.

Others see me as confident and successful, but I'm not.
Have you dedicated your whole adult life to the pursuit of career success, to reaching beyond the glass ceiling? But at what cost?

Often business colleagues see you as confident and successful, but in reality you are shy and lacking in self-esteem. You can still be driven, ambitious and a perfectionist, but with low self-esteem.

To be a high achiever you are often a perfectionist. When you're a perfectionist you are self-critical and do not take criticism well from others. Many high achievers don't feel that they are successful. They are also often the outsiders and feel the need to prove themselves with drive and the relentless pursuit of a goal or challenge. But this pursuit of achievement does not bring happiness, and often it even brings loneliness.

Did you lose your friends, your social life and who you are along the way? Do you live for your work and not work to live? If you were to lose your job or get sick what would you have then? Does it make sense to work that hard if you have no one to share it with, or to talk with about your successes and your failures or discuss those funny moments in your day? It's important to re-evaluate your life every so often and decide if what you're doing is what you *really* want.

Are you happy? You won't know until you try an alternative and you are the only one who can change your situation. And it's never too late to do so. If you can be that successful at work, there is no reason why you can't have as much success with your personal life. It's all about giving yourself a chance.

> *The worst part of success is to try to find someone who is happy for you.*
>
> Bette Midler

They see me as a loser.

Who told you that? No one! (And if they did, should you believe them?) Why do you think that you're a loser? Consider the positive things about yourself (remember the chart you did earlier). Your kindness, your honesty or hard work ethic, or even your best physical assets.

No one is simply just a loser, only in the movies. Yes, life can work against you and everyone has their ups and downs. You may not be the best looking, the most successful, the thinnest or the richest, or you may just have been made redundant or sacked from your job, but that does not make you a loser. Take Frank Spencer in the old TV series *Some Mothers Do 'Ave 'Em*. Whatever he attempted to do always went wrong, but he was endearing, loveable and always well-intentioned and he and his wife Betty really loved each other.

> *No one can make you feel inferior without your consent.*
>
> Eleanor Roosevelt

> *In every aspect of our lives, we are always asking ourselves, "How am I of value?"*
>
> Oprah Winfrey

Are you overly critical of yourself and how others see you?

Are you too harsh on yourself or on in your judgement of others? Maybe you are an only child with the expectancy of being as perfect for your parents as possible. An only child is often the sole focus of their parents' attention and hopes. Only children are usually the highest achievers, perfectionists and over critical of themselves. It's difficult to stop being so self-critical, but if you understand that you don't have to be perfect all the time, life will only become easier.

So who are you?

You may feel differently about yourself tomorrow. We all have a different view and priorities according to what stage of life we are at. Babies expect feeding. Children want to play. Teenagers want sexual experimentation. Young adults think they are immortal. Middle-aged people look back on their youth and wonder where the years went. Everything changes all the time just as you do, so however bad you perceive your life or current situation to be, it will be changing again very soon. I have realised from my own life's highs and lows that bad times will always be replaced by good. Some take longer than others, but they will always come again.

I only see myself as a mum.
Have you forgotten who you are? Do you only see yourself as your children's mum, not as 'you'? And do others, including

your partner, only see you as a mum too, not as that attractive sexy woman you were when you first met (and still are)? Or have you forgotten how to be sexy? Have you forgotten that you have a partner who might find you attractive and would like to interact with you as you once were? Do you find time to do this? It is very important to be able to remember who you are and find time for yourself and also as a partner and lover. However frenetic your life may be, there is always a way (even if it means calling upon your family or friends to help with your kids) to put aside even one night a week to become the old you.

> *Although it's fashionable to complain about the lack of quality family time, more family time can often be the last thing one needs. When it comes to life being "just good enough", sometimes it's the cocktail with the girls and the freedom to push an overpriced lettuce leaf around a large white restaurant plate that makes all the difference.*
>
> Polly Williams
> author of The Rise and Fall of a Yummy Mummy

Bringing up children is never easy and, although always rewarding, it can be emotionally, physically and financially draining. It's easy to become all-consumed by your kids and forget you ever had a life. You may have let yourself go, with the excuses to yourself that you have no time, your children need you 24/7, no one will ever fancy you again or you just aren't interested in men any more. But these are excuses, not reasons to hide away. One day your children will be grown-up and won't need you anymore and then where will you be? Probably feeling lonely and abandoned and wondering where the years went. So it's time to get out of the home and start balancing your life, even if it's only for a few hours a week. You will start to remember what life was like, pre-kids. You could be pleasantly surprised!

I only see myself as my parent's carer.

Do you hanker after freedom and being answerable to no one? To lead a purely selfish self-indulgent life as maybe you once did? But no one can ever be free of dependants of some sort. Parents, in their old age needs, become like your children. It's important to be always there for them, but to keep some time for yourself, even if only for a few hours twice a week in the evening. It's about making a few small rules and boundaries for yourself that you keep to, so you can retain a breathing space for yourself without being suffocated and still give a fulfilled life to both you and your dependants.

Re-invention

Do you believe in yourself? If you believe in yourself, others will. Don't wait for someone else to endorse or confirm your worth. It's all about what messages you give off. Many celebrities and pop stars such as Kylie, Madonna and Lady Gaga are masters of re-invention. Re-invention also helps to keep you feeling and looking younger as you will not be stuck in a rut. You can look older than your biological years by never progressing from that 20 years ago style moment, or equally trying to dress 20 years younger than you are. There is no reason why you can't look a stylish 10 years younger than your real age (see 'Dressing for your age' in Part Two).

There are moments when I can't believe I'm as old as I am, but I feel better physically than I did 10 years ago. I don't think, oh God, I'm missing something.

Madonna

The secret of staying young is to live honestly, eat slowly, and lie about your age.

Lucille Ball

Would you like to look 10 years younger?

*I love walking fast.
That way nobody can see my wrinkles.*

Anita Roddick
founder of The Body Shop

How old do you look? Your biological age? Possibly even older? Would you like to look younger? Looking younger does not need to be created by plastic surgery. It's about your outlook on life, how you carry yourself, stand, speak, and wear your clothes, hair and make-up. Of course plastic surgery can transform, as can non-surgical procedures such as Botox, non-surgical facelifts and peels, but the *inner you* is the one that has to change first.

I feel that I have wasted my life so far and now it's too late.
Do you feel that you are past your sell-by date? Have your best years gone? If Sophia Loren at 70-something can be considered sexy enough to do a photo shoot for Pirelli, then there is hope for all of us that it is never too late to start over.

> *Being 70 is no different from being 69. It's a round number, and there's something about roundness that has always appealed to me.*
>
> Elizabeth Taylor

> *I'm not interested in age. People who tell me their age are silly. You're as old as you feel.*
>
> Elizabeth Arden

I'm thinking about cosmetic surgery.
With all the TV coverage of cosmetic surgery procedures and the trend for thinking that a nip and a tuck can change your life, it's important to realise that actually it won't. Of course bigger bosoms will make you initially more attractive to certain men and a facelift may well take off 10 years, but you are still the same you inside. If you do make these changes, you will need to learn how to adapt to the shift of the perception of you. Many of the TV cosmetic surgery makeover subjects are often rejected by their neighbours and friends

and even partners after the transformation. When the outside persona no longer matches the inside, your old friends and relations may find it hard to equate the new you with the old one. You may find it difficult too. That's why the TV makeover subjects are often offered therapy and counselling after the extreme makeover transformations.

Individuality is beautiful. Old, young, skinny, curvy. I love a face with lines on it. We should work with what we have and make the best of it.

Liv Tyler

When you walk around New York or LA, everyone looks the same. It's pathetic. The lips all look like duck lips, there's no more wrinkles, the noses are all identical, and everything that made someone beautiful has gone. I know what it feels like to think you need to mutilate yourself. I thought, "Maybe if I stick some fake breasts on, it will be OK." But when I hit my sixties I felt so ashamed.

Jane Fonda

Do you ever have any 'you time'?

I have too much to do to look after myself.
If you have too much too do, try to prioritise and focus on the most important things. Maybe some things really don't need to be done today. Maybe you are taking the weight of the world

on your shoulders. Try to delegate, even if it means getting your partner to do something that he would never usually do, and also give small tasks to the children. They may enjoy being given a grown-up seeming job if they are young, and if they are older they could possibly help you more anyway.

Are you trying to be all things to all people? Are you trying to be a good mother, wife, lover, daughter, friend, business woman and more? You may look great from the outside as you look successful, happily married with all material wants and needs satisfied. But are you living on adrenalin, coffee and stress? This is equivalent to running a car on no petrol. You will get ill and then what will happen?

I never have any time for me.
Does everyone always need you? If so, make sure they really can't get hold of you whilst you take some 'you' time doing something that you really enjoy. Maybe it's just watching a TV soap. It doesn't matter what it is if it makes you happy.

Do you often feel alone, even when you're surrounded by people? Do you keep yourself so busy that you don't have to think about what's wrong in your life or your needs? Life is different now from how it was 50 years ago. It's faster paced and fewer people live within a community or with a family support system around them. Many of us have relocated for that better job, or as a result of a marriage break-up, and can feel very isolated. When you are alone (and you can feel alone even if you have children whom you are close to, as you need adult company too), you can immerse yourself in your job or your children with

47

no 'you time'. But you need 'down time' to concentrate on your wants and needs and re-energising yourself.

This time will enable you to escape from the treadmill of your everyday life and give you a break, even if only once or twice a week. It could be something simple and mundane, or as far removed from your real life as you like, even if it seems mad to you at first. It could be something you always wanted to do. Maybe vary your days, take a different method of transport to work, take time for a quick coffee/gossip with a girlfriend, or stop off after work for a drink somewhere you've never been before with a work colleague. You never know who you could meet or what could happen. It could be fun!

Some suggestions:
- Read a new book or a magazine
- Learn to play a musical instrument
- Singing lessons
- Join the local amateur dramatic society
- An at DIY home beauty or spa style treatment, even give yourself a proper manicure or pedicure
- Take a walk
- Look in a cook book and try cooking a new dish, or even a cake
- Go on a window shopping expedition
- Try a yoga class or DVD
- Get a dog. You'll *have* to take time out for both yourself and the dog to walk it twice a day and you will get exercise into the bargain.

I feel guilty and selfish putting myself first.

Do you feel guilty putting yourself first? This is normal, especially when you emerge from a long term relationship. Do you only feel worthwhile when you feel needed? But being needed isn't the same thing as being loved... Do you feel yourself repeating patterns whereby you are attracted to needy and childlike men? Do you try to feel better in yourself and gain self-esteem by giving in to their needs and demands and trying to make them feel better? You must be responsible for your own feelings and they must be responsible for theirs. You are an independent adult, not an emotional prop. Although, if you do care mutually for someone, then the relationship should be a two-way street where you both offer support to each other but neither becomes a crutch.

How you care about yourself determines the quality of your life. You need to put yourself first to have enough energy to care for others. Even an occasional 10 minute time out for yourself will help improve your quality of life. By being good to yourself, you can bring out the best in others.

I feel guilty when I sit down to relax.

You need to recharge your batteries, otherwise you will be irritable, feel constantly tired, forgetful and crave foods that give you a quick fix of energy. Slow down, you only have one life. If you do slow down, you might find you can prioritise and find those things that are truly important to you.

> *If there's no inner peace, people can't give it to you. The husband can't give it to you. Your children can't give it to you. You have to give it to you.*
>
> Linda Evans

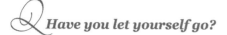 *Have you let yourself go?*

I've no time or no money.

Do you neglect your personal grooming because you don't have time or money, or because you don't feel a need as there is no one else to see you? Grooming and keeping your body in the best shape possible will make you feel your best. Just because you may not have a boyfriend doesn't mean that you don't need to shave your legs, or have a bikini wax. Hair colour should be kept up, with roots being re-touched and a haircut to suit your age and face shape. If money is short, choose a colour and cut that are low-maintenance. Looking good is all about feeling good from the inside, and that means that you should feel good about your whole body under the covering of clothes in the same way as a sexy set of underwear will make you feel sexier even if no one else sees them.

I've had a serious illness and have lost the incentive to look good anymore.

How do you come to terms with a life-threatening disease such as cancer that can leave your family and loved ones on their own? If the disease is caught early enough, together with a positive attitude and the best medical treatment, how do you feel once in remission? Do you feel that others treat you differently when you only want to be treated the same as you were before?

Even if it appears on the outside that you have everything to live for, together with the support of a loving family, it doesn't mean that you feel the same way about yourself inside, despite having been granted that precious second chance of life. You may feel that having faced the possibility of death, thinking about how you look is totally shallow. You may feel that no one will ever fancy you anyway, post breast cancer mastectomy. But it's important to remember that looking good is part of being alive and feeling good.

You owe it to both yourself and your partner and family to look your best, now that you are feeling well and are well. Why dwell in the past? Look forward. Why not feel proud of yourself for conquering the disease and also feel proud of yourself for how you now look too? There are many celebrities who have come through breast cancer and are brave enough to re-appear in the public eye, both during and post treatment. It's great that they do as it shows a great example of courage and how to still hold your head up high and look good in the face of adversity. You will give yourself back your self –esteem when you feel good and both you and your family will benefit. Face the world and take it on.

I had a serious accident and I feel that my life has come to an end due to the scarring.

Do you really feel that your life has come to a full stop? Do you think that new friends will only see your disfigurement or scarring? And what will your old friends say or do? They may be initially cautious and shy about what to say to you, but will accept you in the same way as they knew you before, as they will only see the old you. Maybe your confidence will have taken a knock, but now it's even more important to concentrate on using that power of attraction, of using your personality and charisma, drawing their eyes and attention to the best parts of you. In that way your new friends will be drawn to you whatever your disability.

> *I don't look too bad for someone my age, with my history of illnesses and operations and all those anaesthetics. When they knock you out, it gives you time to catch up on your beauty sleep.*
>
> Elizabeth Taylor

Everything has gone downhill since I reached the menopause.

With what do we associate women's menopausal symptoms – a cougar with a toy boy boyfriend, or is it hot sweats, flushes and an apple-shaped middle-aged spread for most of us? Do you now think that half your life is now past and that youth is behind you? Since 50 is the new 40 there is no reason why being menopausal or post-menopausal should mean a major life change. At least you shouldn't have to worry about birth control anymore, so sex should be more enticing, not less. Nowadays with the correct nutrition, and hormonal support if necessary, most women should be able to breeze through with few symptoms. There should be no reason not to let yourself go.

You may have found that your body has become more curvaceous, with more flesh mostly in the wrong places, but you may also have a bigger bust. So why not look at the bright side. This could be the first time you've had a bust since you were pregnant!

I have passed my best years.
There is something positive to be gained and enjoyed from each period of your life. Yes, you may not look so youthful any more but look at the knowledge and experience you now have. You will attract admirers with your aura, personality and conversation as much as superficial youth and beauty. 50-somethings like Twiggy, 60-somethings like Helen Mirren and 70-pluses like Lauren Bacall all look wonderful and are ambassadors for how to look stunning for their age. Yes, they are celebrities, with the money and access to the best beauty and style advisors and therapists but they have all been through the menopause too. Everyone, however famous, has the same bodily functions. So look forward to the next part of your life.

> *If I could go back in a time machine and talk to myself aged 25, I'd say this "Don't waste your time on being shy. Don't let anyone sap your self-esteem. You're beautiful, intelligent and talented, so don't let the bastards get you down."*
>
> Joan Collins

Q Now that you have journeyed through the first stage of questions about how you feel about yourself, how would you like to change?

I would like to be more assertive, and more confident.
I would like to look more stylish and look better.
I would like to get a new life.

You can have all this, as you create your own destiny. Things don't just happen. You have to make them happen.

So how do you do that?

Don't be one of life's victims. Be proactive and make small changes step by step.

Create a mental picture of the new you that you would like to be in, say, a year's time and then in a few more years' time. Imagine that 'new you' living the life you would like and being that person you never thought you could be. But it has to be achievable, don't be unrealistic. Then it will actually work.

In Part Two of the journey you can find out how you can change the physical you, with clothes, beauty and make-up tips, healthy eating and exercise.

*Vitality shows in not only the ability
to persist but the ability to start over.*

Scott Fitzgerald

*The key to realizing a dream is to focus not on success
but on significance – and then even the small steps and
little victories along your path with take on greater
meaning.*

Oprah Winfrey

Part Two

The Outer You

● ●

How you can change yourself physically

The second stage of the journey to the new you

> *Right now you are one choice away from a new beginning – one that leads you toward becoming the fullest human being you can be.*
>
> Oprah Winfrey

Now that we have looked at how you feel about yourself, what would you like to start changing about yourself?

This section covers how you can change any part of the *physical* you from top to toe, using my celebrity beauty, fashion, make-up and exercise tips and some suggestions of non-surgical beauty procedures.

You will be able to find out how you can change or improve your problem areas, but most importantly, come to terms with whatever shape you actually are. Imagine I am with you in your home, talking about you and your life. We have discussed how you feel about yourself and how you feel others perceive you. Now we are going to talk about looking your physical best.

How would you like to be perceived on first impression? All it takes is 30 seconds for someone to make an initial judgement of you, so first impressions are important. A first impression is what you give off overall – a combination of your personality, confidence, posture, body language, voice, eye contact, and also hair, make-up, clothes, accessories. The mix of the inner and outer you gives someone a way of assessing you, before getting to know you properly.

The outer you is as important as the inner you, as it is part of what makes you unique. So let's start with making the best of the outer you. We will start at the head and work down to your toes!

Face

Men become much more attractive when they start looking older. But it doesn't do much for women, though we do have an advantage: make-up.

Bette Davis

Most of the celebrities I have styled over the years have had top make-up artists working with them to help them look their absolute best. Celebrities, like all of us, have their 'feeling ugly' days with bad skin moments, major spot outbreaks, puffy eyes, dark shadows, skin allergies and more. But the final images we see of them are of flawless perfection, due to the expertise of make-up artists and also the wizardry of the magazine art department with digital re-touching. So we tend to forget that even celebrities are human and however beautiful they are, their imperfections need covering up with make-up just as ours do.

The celebrity has to have absolute trust in both the make-up artist and the stylist (myself) to create an image that gives her confidence and makes her feel transformed from her own inner perception of an ugly duckling to her public image of the beautiful swan. You would not believe how many celebrities have major insecurities and confidence crises before appearing in public or in front of a camera. To look beautiful you have to feel beautiful, as beauty begins within.

> *Beauty is not an easy thing to live with. Often the most beautiful people are the most self-conscious.*
> Sarah Doukas, Storm modelling agency

According to a survey of 5,000 women, only one in 20 feel confident without make-up. As many as 80 per cent said you don't leave home without wearing it, mostly because you believe it makes you look sexier and feel 'happier with life'. Another survey reported that women in the workplace are more successful when wearing makeup. In my opinion this is because the first impressions of a woman wearing a small amount of well-applied makeup says 'well- groomed, takes pride in her appearance and therefore pride in her job too'.

> *I'd asked my mother what she did in the war when her flat had been blown up. She remembered taking a bottle of Shocking perfume, by Schiaparelli. She said, "When there's nothing left, you stick to the superfluous".*
>
> Jane Birkin

Buying make-up and the anticipation of putting it on can make you feel good. You can wake up looking and feeling rough and, even with a minimal application of products, you can become an improved you in less than five minutes.

Creating a make-up look is a gradual build-up of effect. Each item will have its own job to do, but will balance another. Doing make-up is like decorating a room. You have to prime the walls and fill the cracks before painting. Once you have the whole room painted uniformly, then you can start adding the furniture and colour touches with cushions, curtains and accessories. Each time you add a chair or a cushion you need to stand back and look at how it affects the balance and proportions of the room space. In the same way, the foundation is your blank wall with the concealer and cover-up being your 'fillers'. The eye shadow and blusher and lipstick will create light and shade, and the balance and intensity of how you apply each one will make a difference to how the shape of your face and features appear.

How do you know your face shape?

Look in the mirror and pull back all your hair from your face. Do not wear any clothing that clutters up your neckline. A towel wrapped round you, leaving your shoulders bare, is best.

Use a lipstick, or crayon or something that is easily wiped from the mirror. Standing very close up to the mirror, draw the outline of your face on the mirror in front of you.

Be honest and critical with yourself to decide if you have any other prominent features such as a high forehead, long nose or receding chin.

Once you have accepted your features you can disguise and balance them with your make-up and hairstyle.

Eyebrows

Before you start your make-up, you need to look closely at your eyebrows. When did you last consider what they looked like? Have you plucked them recently or did you over-pluck them years ago? What shape are they? Could they be improved? Or don't you care as you think they don't make a difference?

Plucking your eyebrows will open up your eyes and take ten years off your face. Eyebrows frame your eyes. Your eyes are the first thing that most people notice and are the 'front door' to your 'visible' emotions. So it is very important that your eyebrows are well groomed and plucked to work best for your face and eye shape. Your eyebrow shape can make your eyes appear more open, seem larger or smaller and completely change your whole facial look. If you look at many celebrity eyebrows, you will find that as the celebrities have become more high profile and groomed, all have undergone an eyebrow makeover from heavy, thick brows to finer, groomed and contoured brows (think Liz Hurley from before wearing that life changing 'safety pin' red carpet dress to how she looks now).

Do you know how to shape your brows?

I don't know where to start plucking from.
Your eyebrow shape will define your eyes. They should be gently arched and taper away. To find out exactly where the brows should start and end, you should hold a pencil or make-up brush vertically alongside your nose. Your inside brow edge should start at the point where the pencil meets it. The brow arch should be somewhere directly above your iris. The outer brow edge should ideally be at the point where your pencil creates an angled line from your nose past the edge of your eye to your brow edge. You should never pluck from above your eyebrows. Only pluck from beneath (in bright light, so you can see what you're doing), tweezing a hair at a time, whilst checking in the mirror how this step-by-step removal is altering your brow shape. You don't want to end up with pencil-thin brows or over-rounded brows. To help you see the shape you would like to achieve, brush your

eyebrows upwards into the shape you would like them to be, and then pencil in the actual shape you want. That way you can see where to pluck and not to pluck.

It hurts.
It's best to pluck after a warm shower or bath as your pores will be open. Always pluck in the direction the hairs are growing.

Can I use any other method?
You can go to a salon to have your eyebrows shaped by threading. This is where hairs are removed one at a time with a tiny thread. You can also have them waxed. There are also brow-shaping stencil kits you can buy that can help you make sure that your brow shape ends up being one that you wanted and that suits your face shape.

What shape is good for my face shape?
If you have close set eyes and you want to make them appear further apart, then lightly extend the brows further outward. Eyes with a deep socket can take eyebrows that are slightly thicker. Eyes with only a little space between eye and brow need as much space as possible to open them up.

My face shape is oval.
Try to pluck the brows so they
taper and slant upwards towards the temples. Take the
most hairs away from underneath the outer edges. The
shape should compliment your
face shape.

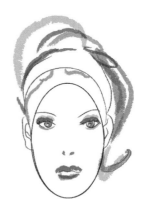

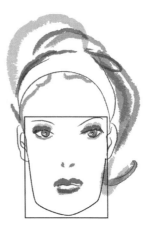

My face shape is square.
Your eyebrows should soften
your wide face shape with a
gentle arch. As you have a
strong face shape, you can
take heavier eyebrows, so don't
over-pluck.

My face shape is rectangular.
As you want to widen your long
face, you should keep your eyebrows strong but well-shaped,
balancing out your square jaw
line.

My face shape is an inverted triangle.

As your face shape is wide on the forehead with high cheek-bones, you want to have gently arched eyebrows which do not appear to make your upper face even wider. So keep them well groomed and well plucked. Only the stronger face shapes can take heavier eyebrows.

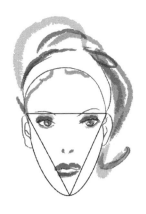

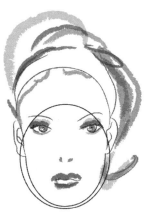

My face shape is round.

You want to balance the roundness of your face with straighter lines. So when you pluck your eyebrows try to make them less curved taper-ing away to a slim line at the outer edges.

Best tweezers

A good, gripping pair of tweezers is essential to remove those stray brow hairs. The best, used by most celebrity make-up artists and myself, are by Tweezerman. Of course there are many excellent high street brands too.

I have over-plucked over the years and my eyebrows now won't grow back.

Once you have over plucked, especially over many years, you can't turn the clock back, but you can try to do some damage limitation. With over-plucked eyebrows you will need to fill in where you would like the thicker eyebrow to be. You can use a natural shade of powder shadow with a chisel shaped brush or an eyebrow pencil. It is easiest to create a natural looking brow with brush and powder, using little, feathery brush strokes, but pencil may last longer in place.

There is nothing you can do to make hairs grow back, but if you want to do something permanently instead of using make-up, you can have eyebrows tattooed. You don't visit a tattoo parlour but a semi-permanent make-up artist or salon where they specialise in semi-permanent make-up procedures. The missing eyebrows are tattooed on in feathery strokes. This will last around 18 months.

The eyebrows must be made to look natural – not too dark or too 'one-line'.

How can I keep my eyebrows tamed? They always look unruly.

You can brush them into shape with an old, clean tooth brush or cleaned up old mascara wand. Once brushed into shape, you can use a clear mascara or brow gel to set them. If there is a stray, longer hair, you could trim it with nail scissors.

My eyebrows look so blonde they disappear.

You could tint your brows with a light grey-brown eyelash

tint. You can do this at home or at a beauty salon. This works very well and lasts around six weeks. Or you could use a powder shadow or pencil to emphasise your brows.

There are plenty of tools and products you can get your hands on for taming those eyebrows, including an old toothbrush, an eyebrow pencil, and an eyebrow kit.

Make-up

So now that your eyebrows have been groomed and shaped, you can start on your make-up.

Everyone looks better with some make-up, especially as you get older. I meet so many women who tell me that they have never worn any and don't know how to apply it. Applying your daily make-up should be something that is as familiar to you as brushing your teeth. Once you've put on your make up, you should be able to forget about it. It's not necessary to cake it on: less is *always* more.

It should be applied lightly and not be noticeable, especially during the daytime. It should enhance and draw attention to your best features, and can be used to make small eyes bigger, close-set eyes further apart, thin lips fuller, cheeks more contoured, nose more chiselled, and conceal under-eye shadows. It can help you look less tired, younger, fresher and certainly more groomed.

Decide how much time you have before you start your make-up as that will dictate how far you can go with your chosen look. You may have five minutes before the school run or before you go to work, but an hour before a party. Never experiment with make-up before you are about to go out. Save this for an evening in when you can remove it again if it doesn't work! There is no point putting on your best outfit for work or for a party unless you 'finish' the look. The finish is about the make-up as much as a stylish bag and shoes. It should be *you* that people are looking at, not what you are wearing.

Why don't you wear make-up?

Why should I change the habits of a lifetime?
Because you are embarking on a step-by-step journey to discovering the 'new you'. You will never know if something works for you until you try.

I feel make-up is unnecessary.
Everyone needs *some* make-up. Ok... maybe not *everyone* needs some makeup, but you will certainly look an even better

version of yourself with some, even if you feel good without it. Any one of the following can make a difference: concealer, blusher, a single application of mascara, or a hint of lip gloss.

I might look silly.
You won't look silly if you apply less rather than more, and apply it correctly with colours that work for your skin tone and age, which we'll consider later. People will notice you look healthy and well – not notice that you are wearing make-up.

I think that anything more than some mascara or lipstick is overkill.
Then just wear those. There are no rules about what make-up you should or shouldn't wear. You have to feel comfortable and still feel like 'you'.

> *The eyebrow pencil and false eyelashes were essential; my mother (Judy Garland) didn't feel dressed without them.*
>
> Lorna Luft

I don't know what products to buy.
Start off with the basic ones. You don't have to go for the most expensive. Very often factories that produce for top end cosmetic companies manufacture for the high street brands as well. Start with mascara, neutral coloured eye shadows, maybe in a lighter and a darker grey or a lighter and a darker brown, a foundation that suits your skin type, some lip gloss

and some blusher. Good soft bristle brushes are very important, not the token miniature sized ones that accompany the products.

I don't know how to apply it.
Make-up is about enhancing your best features and detracting from your worst. Make-up should not be noticeable or too heavy, unless you are a model in a fashion or beauty photography shoot or on TV. You can learn how to apply simple, daily make-up from this book by following my step-by-step instructions. It's not hard and once you have had some practice your make-up routine can be quick and easy. You will wonder how you lived without using it at all. More glamorous evening make-up will take longer to experiment with. But it's like riding a bicycle. Once you have mastered it, you will never forget.

My make-up has been the same for the last 20 years.
Foundation badly applied, thickly plastered, wrong colour (too dark, to orange or too pink) will add years on to you. Also lipstick that is too red or too vibrant, whether pink or coral, will do no favours for older women. In all cases less is more. The key words to good make-up application are blend, blend and blend.

Make-up brushes
To apply make-up well you need proper brushes. Ideally, you need a selection. At least one for eye shadow, but a few would be better so that you can have one for each colour you use.

These should be quite flat and easy to manipulate around the eye contours. Brushes for powder blusher and powder should be soft and largish. The eyebrow brush can be chisel shaped; I find that shape the easiest to use. Lip brushes are small and pointed. You can buy natural bristle brushes at art shops and many celebrity make-up artists now create their own ranges of make-up and brushes at high street prices.

When did you last update your make-up bag?

When I ask my clients to show me their make-up bags, many show me ones with contents well past their sell-by date that have been languishing at the bottom of the bag since they started wearing make-up: lipsticks with no lipstick left in the barrel; colours that no longer suit their skin tones or hair colouring; tired 'free with the product' mini-brushes and sponge applicators; dried up, gunky mascaras. It's important to update your make-up regularly.

Why do I need to update my make-up? I hardly ever wear it. Most beauty products only have a shelf life of around six months. You may notice that your lipsticks and foundations begin to smell stale after too many months.

As you age, your skin tones change along with your hair colour and you will find that those products that you have had forever no longer suit you. You may also need to change your make-up style to be appropriate to your age. (We'll talk about this later.)

> *You wouldn't recognise me from photographs 20 years ago. I feel you change every 12 years.*
>
> Francesca Annis

Q Do you know how to adapt your make-up to your age?

Are you stuck in a make-up time warp? More mature skins with wrinkles and crow's feet need foundations that have light reflective qualities. Matte eye shadows are better than shiny and anything glittery or pearlised is really not very flattering for more mature skin.

> *What's wrong with having lines around your eyes, anyway? I actually like them... if you want to look better, get a new hairdo and learn how to do your make-up properly.*
>
> Make-up artist Bobbi Brown

Q Do you have no time in the morning to put on any make-up?

Everyone can use a little help, however beautiful they are, and how long can it take to put on a little mascara and some lip gloss? You need to find a make-up routine that suits your daily routine.

If people think I look good, it's the make-up.

Francesca Annis

I'm always late!

Maybe you don't want to wear a foundation, but you could try a tinted moisturiser, which will moisturise and give you a healthy glow. It only takes a few minutes to apply and is two products in one application, saving time! Instead of wearing mascara, have you considered dyeing your eyelashes? It saves you having to put mascara on each day.

I have to get the children ready for school.

Blusher always helps you look healthier and gives your cheeks some shape whilst lip gloss adds that extra finishing touch. Why can't you feel good about yourself, even if you're on the school run? It could only take an extra five minutes in your getting up and out routine. If you're a newly single mum, you never know who you could meet outside the school gates... there may be some newly single dads out there too.

I have to leave too early for work.

If you deal with clients or customers face to face, how you look will be associated with a perception of the brand you represent. So however smart your clothes may be, it is important to wear some make-up as it will make you look not only healthier but better groomed and more polished.

Q How do you adapt your make-up to your face shape?

(See 'How to find your face shape' section)

How you apply your make-up will affect the look of your face shape. So you can use blusher, shading, highlights and eye shadow to create contours and the impression of better balanced features. To highlight, you can use a 'highlighter' powder, cream or pencil that is similar to a neutral pale shiny eye shadow or a light reflective product.

I have a round face.

Use light and shade to create contours. Apply your blusher onto the apples of your cheeks (the fleshy front area) keeping the colour inwards rather than outwards.

I have a narrow face.

Use blusher to draw the eye outwards, applying the blusher less centrally, more toward the cheekbones.

I have a square face.

Use light and shade as you would with a round face shape. Apply the blusher to the apples of the cheeks.

I have a double chin.

Use a browny shade of blusher *subtly* under the jaw line (but make sure there are no tide marks). The shading will draw attention away from the chin. Blusher and highlighter will attract attention to the eye area and the cheekbones.

I have a wide nose.
You can shade down either side of the nose with a browny shade of blusher. Be minimal – you don't want to look as though you have bruises.

I have a long nose.
You can shade *under* the tip of the nose and highlight down the centre.

I have close set eyes.
Take your eye shadow shading further out than usual. Use a lighter shade of shadow on the inner part of your lid whilst the darker shade and shading should be toward the outer edge. Eyeliner can start from the centre of your eyelash line on your upper lid to slightly outside your eye edge.

I have wide set eyes.
Apply your eye shadow colour more centrally and in a more rounded way on your eyelid and into the socket, rather than taking the colour outwards. You can use your paler shadow on the central part of the lid if you like, with the deeper shade into the whole socket-not just the outer edge. You can take the eyeliner all the way along the eyelash line on the top lid from the inside corner, but stopping the line short at the outer edge.

I have small eyes.

Never use liner on the upper lid, or a dark shadow as under-eyeliner as this will close up your eye. Use a darker shadow in the socket to lengthen outwards, and from the mid to outer eyelash edge to lengthen outwards, with lots of mascara mostly on the upper outer lashes.

I have a high forehead.

Use a matte powder bronzer or a brownish toned blusher horizontally along the top of your forehead, to help give the appearance of a lower forehead. The shading will help create an impression of this.

I have a wide forehead.

Use the matte bronzer powder or brownish toned blusher vertically down the temples, to help give the appearance of a narrower forehead. The shading will again help create this impression.

I would like Kate Moss style cheekbones.

Use your blusher not only on the apples of your cheeks but in a more lengthy and diagonal way.

I always look shiny even if I keep powdering.

You can try using an oil-absorbing under-foundation product to stop greasiness before you apply your make-up.

Sometimes my skin looks tired whatever moisturiser I use.
You can try a primer or illuminator, after your moisturiser and before you apply your makeup. A primer helps even out skin tone, create a smooth surface for foundation and give a radiant glow. An illuminator will give you an instantly fresher look.

Foundation

The most important element of your make-up is foundation which serves to even out your skin tones, allowing the rest of your make-up to create highlights and shadows. Foundation should be applied to be invisible. It should match your skin tone and even out any irregularities of colouration, pigmentation and blemishes. It should be applied with your fingertips or a small make-up sponge to achieve even coverage. When applying your foundation, always make sure that it is blended out at the jaw line and the neck.

Never, ever try foundation colours on the back of your hand. The correct place is at the bottom of your cheek near your jaw line. This is where your foundation should blend and match your skin tone. When shopping for your foundation, you will not be able to see the true colour of the foundation unless you take yourself and a mirror out of the store and into the daylight as the lighting inside shops can be misleading.

Triangular sponges

These small make-up sponges are used to apply foundation more subtly, smoothly and evenly. They can be dampened before use to lessen make-up 'tide marks' and caked make-up. You can buy them in most high street chemists.

Light-reflecting foundations

You can help diminish the look of fine lines and wrinkles with light-reflecting foundations.

There are many choices of brand in all price ranges. You may find that some suit your skin type better than others

My skin feels dry when I wear foundation.

If your skin feels too dry when you wear foundation, you could try adding a touch of your daily moisturiser when you apply it. Or you can choose a foundation that has extra hydrating properties; these are often marketed for more mature skins.

My make-up always settles into my surrounding eye wrinkles.

Buy a foundation that is advertised to be suited to more mature skins and that is also light reflective. Don't use a heavy foundation and powder, especially around the eye area. Blend it away before you reach the surrounding eye lines. Be minimal with face powder as it's the powder that tends to sit in the wrinkles. Keep to only powdering the t- zone of forehead and nose and chin, or you could try blotting papers instead of powder (see "Powders and Blotting Papers").

Spray foundation/Air brush foundation

This foundation gives an even natural look. It is often used on TV presenters' faces to give a sheer, even look, as high definition TV shows every blemish and flaw.

I have facial hair and when I wear foundation it emphasises the hairs.

Just as a wall needs smoothing, sanding and preparing before painting, so does your face before you apply makeup. If you have superfluous facial hair, either on the lips or at the sides of your face, it is important to remove it. Especially as you reach the menopause, as you may find odd hairs sprouting up where there weren't ones before.

If you bleach your facial hair, it will become less noticeable, but when you add foundation, the make-up will sit on the hairs, making them more visible. You should look into laser removal or electrolysis to help decrease your hair. Laser, although much more expensive, is quicker and less painful (see non-surgical procedures). Never, ever shave. You will end up with bristles like a man (see section on hair removal).

But I really don't like the feeling of make-up on my skin.

Make-up should not feel heavy on the skin and certainly not look as if it is caked on. If you wear a foundation, it should not be visible but only be there to even out your complexion. You could try a tinted moisturiser if you prefer an even more natural look and feel.

Tinted moisturiser

These moisturisers can be used instead of foundation as they will still give some cover whilst also giving a healthy, *slightly* tanned glow. We are not talking orange here or shades darker!

Powder

So, should you powder your face?

A light dusting of powder can be used to fix make-up straight after application (with a large soft brush or velvety powder puff pad) or to blot away shine later in the day. It should not be used liberally. Less is always more, especially around the eyes as powder can sit in your wrinkles if over-zealously applied.

I always look shiny after an hour or so.

Always carry a pack of blotting papers with you. They are a great way to remove excess shine as they will blot the greasy areas instead of creating a build up of powder.

Bronzers

I would like to look browner.

Foundation should not make you appear suntanned or darker. That is the job of a bronzing powder. With a dusting of a bronzing powder you can look natural and healthy throughout the year. A bronzer gives a subtle golden glow and is great for using both on the face and the décolleté. You do not apply a bronzer all over the face, just where the sun might naturally increase colour. Good makeup is about looking natural.

Self tan for the face

I would like a more permanent facial tan.

A fake tan for the face needs to be applied evenly as it does not wash off. To apply more subtly, moisturise before applying the self-tanning product..

Concealer

I have dark under-eye shadows. If I cover them with foundation then I look even more crinkly around the eyes.

Use a concealer, not your foundation base, to freshen and rejuvenate skin and lighten any under-eye dark shadows or lines, and nose to mouth lines. Apply with a brush and blend away with the brush or with light tapping movements of your finger.

A concealer is a key product to have in your make-up bag. A concealer contains light reflective properties that help disguise dark eye shadows and lines. You apply them after you have put on your foundation. This is *the* product that will make you look instantly younger and refreshed.

My age spots and blemishes still show under my foundation.

You can't hide blemishes or age spots with your foundation as you'll end up with a caked mask. So try using a warm-toned concealer or spot cover, applied with a small brush onto the small problem areas after applying your foundation. There are also specific creams and products that can help to fade age spots with regular use.

Spot cover up

This is for specifically targeting and covering blemishes. One shade paler than your skin is best. You can apply these before or after your foundation. But I find that application after foundation is better, as you can then blend away the cover up more effectively.

Camouflage make-up

This is designed for extra coverage to conceal acne, vitiligo, rosacea and burns. It can be fantastic in helping to create a flawless complexion. There are specialist websites and professional make up shops that sell camouflage makeup.

Blusher

Cream blusher can be applied with your fingertips or a medium-sized, flat brush. It is more difficult to apply than a powder blusher, as the edges of the blusher area must be blended away.

Powder blusher is the most commonly used blusher and works well for all skin types and ages. Less is always more with all make-up. Powder blusher is applied with a larger soft brush with small circular motions. Cream blusher will give your cheeks more of a glow, whilst powder blusher colour will give more depth of colour.

Mousse blusher is long lasting and feels wonderfully light. It should be applied with your fingertip and then blended away. It looks natural and fresh. You can wear it over your moisturiser or your foundation.

Lip and cheek stain is a handy handbag/holiday multi-use product that can be used on both lips and cheeks. It' is important to blend well on cheeks.

I don't know where to put the blusher.
Look in the mirror and smile whilst applying the blusher to the apple of your cheeks. Blusher should be subtly applied to the apples of the cheeks, not below (the apples being the fleshy front area of your cheeks, not your cheekbones). You never want your cheek colour to be a *noticeable* daub. It should just be giving you a healthier rosier hue. You don't want to look like Coco the clown. If you have any spots in the area where you may be placing the blusher, apply powder over the concealer before you apply the blusher, unless you are using a cream blusher.

Highlighter will highlight the area you apply it to. So if you wish to accentuate your cheekbones or brow bones this is the product for you.

Eye shadow
Eye shadow should be applied with a good, soft, natural, long-handled paintbrush style brush, and always be blended away, leaving no hard lines. It is impossible to achieve this with the

83

free sponge applicators that come with the eye shadows. Using light and shade, eye shadow can be used to change the appearance of your eye shape (see make-up for your face shape).

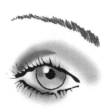 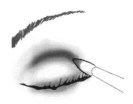

My eye shadow never stays put, but slides into the creases.
The trick is to put foundation over the eyelids first, then apply powder eye shadow.

My lids are now droopy with no defined socket.
With droopy eyelids it is very important not to let the eye-shadow sink into the skin folds. Gently lift each eyebrow with your finger, so that you can see the socket area more clearly and make it easier to apply the shadow. Keep the colour on the lid paler and darker in the socket, to give the illusion of a still existing socket definition.

Eyeliner pencils/kohl
To add extra intensity and definition to your eye make-up you can use eyeliners or kohl.

Eyeliner pencils are nice and soft, don't drag on the eye, and last well. You can use them along the upper lid lash line, or inside the bottom lid edge. Kohl can be used in the same way as it usually comes in pencil form too. It can have a softer and smudgier effect than eye pencils. If you want a natural effect that accentuates the eye, then use a brown or black. If you want to follow a seasonal fashion trend, then you can use colours such as blue or green or a metallic. Using waterproof eyeliner on the bottom inner lid will help its staying power throughout the day.

Liquid eyeliner

You may prefer liquid liner, as it can give a more defined line than the smudgy or softer effect of pencils or kohl pencils. Use black or colour for enhancing the lash line. You could extend the line beyond the eye to lengthen the appearance of your eyes, or give a 50s outer edge flick.

Eyelashes

Eyelash curlers

Use eyelash curlers before you apply your mascara or false lashes. You can also buy heated eyelash curlers. These can be more effective instantly, in the same way as heated rollers or curling tongs are when creating a curly hair style. Eyelash curlers open up your eyes and make your lashes look so much longer. Be careful not to use heated eyelash curlers daily as they can weaken your lashes.

Mascara

Apply your mascara from under the base of the lashes to the tips. Start at the centre of the lashes, then work to the inner and outer edge (or whichever way is comfortable for you). Then repeat the application from above the lashes. When you apply the mascara to the bottom lashes, make sure you don't get the mascara onto your skin. If you do make a mistake, remove the spot with a cotton bud. It's easier to put mascara on the top lashes when you raise your head and look down the tip of your nose: it helps stop your newly wet lashes brushing your lids.

If you are short sighted, and you don't wear contact lenses, but do wear specs, you may find it easier to apply your makeup in a magnifying mirror, or to buy specs that have lenses that fold down individually for ease of makeup application.

Mascara gives the finishing touch to your eye make-up. You can add less or more according to whether you are going for a natural daytime or full on party make-up.

Mascara should not be gunky, heavy or cloggy when applied, especially when it is for daytime wear. Brown mascara can often be more flattering than black if you are fair-haired and fair-skinned. Mascara can simply add colour or can add volume with lash-lengthening filaments.

Cotton buds

These are great for cleaning up those accidental smudges of mascara, and tidying up hard eye shadow edges which should always be blended away.

My mascara always ends up smudged around my eyes.
You could try a good waterproof or smudge-proof mascara, even if you aren't on the beach. If you are a bride, likely to be teary or emotional, at a party getting hot and sweaty, or caught in the rain, there is nothing worse than having mascara running down your cheeks. You will need a special waterproof oil-based mascara remover to remove this mascara with ease. Your eyes are precious and should be treated with gentleness. Tugging and pulling will instantly age your skin around your eyes.

I don't like the feel of mascara
Why not try having your eyelashes tinted, if you don't like wearing mascara. You can also do this yourself at home. If you want to wake up looking as glamorous as you did the night before, there is also the option of lash extensions that can be applied professionally at salons. These will last for a few months, and will fall out naturally together with your own lashes' monthly growing cycle. Never try to remove lash extensions yourself. You will be pulling out your natural lashes at the same time!

False Lashes

How do I apply false lashes?

Begin by curling your own eyelashes with your eyelash curlers. Put a tiny bit of glue along the band of the eyelashes. False eyelashes with a clear band may look better on than those with a black band, especially if you are a novice eyelash applier. This is because the base of the false lashes is less visible, so any imperfections that occur during application will be less noticed. Leave the glue to dry until it's tacky rather than wet. Using tweezers, place the eyelashes on the eye line. Do not leave a gap. You can use a liquid eyeliner after you have stuck on the lashes. It can cover up any mistakes. Finish off with a coat of mascara which is the key to blending your fake and natural lashes together.

Vaseline

This can be used on eyelashes, brows and lips. This not only nourishes your lashes, but gives them a glossy natural look. It helps set your eyebrows. It moisturises your lips.

Lips

Lip liners

Lip liner should not show. If you do use it, it should be as close a shade as possible to your own lips. It is used to re-shape or even out the lip line, ready for infill by smudging more of the lip liner within the new line and then adding lipstick or lip gloss.

My lipstick always bleeds into the lines around my lips.
To stop your lipstick bleeding into those feather lines around
the lip line, set the lipstick colour. Put a tissue between your
lips and gently close them onto the freshly applied lipstick to
soak up the excess.

Lipstick and lip gloss

Lipsticks come both matte (not shiny) and glossy. Some
lipsticks have moisturisers added and vitamins A and E;
others can be extra long-lasting (up to five hours).

Lipstick needs more precision in its application, whereas
lip gloss can be applied without a mirror if needs be. Lip gloss
often now has added ingredients that encourage the blood
flow in the lips and give a short-term plumping effect with a
bit of a sexy tingle on application.

Do you know how to transform your
daytime make-up into night-time make-up?

I work late and have to go out for the evening straight
from work.
With no time to wash your face before going out, you can re-
moisturise (especially around the eye area); touch up with
concealer to hide your under-eye shadows, and re-apply blusher.
You can add to your eye shadow and re-apply your eyeliner. You
can go much darker for the evening. Add masses of mascara and
finally lip gloss. This should take no more than five minutes.

I don't know how to make my everyday make-up more glamorous for a party.

An evening make-up can be darker and smokier around the eyes and have a stronger coloured lipstick than day time, but it is best to *either* have dark, smoky eyes and natural coloured lips *or* strong coloured lips and natural eyes. Never the two, as you will look over made up. There is a fine line between over made up and a sexy glamorous make-up.

> *When it comes to make-up, my message is, be yourself and let yourself be seen. Don't slosh so much make-up on that you can't see the real person.*
>
> Julie Andrews

Eye care

Looking after your eyes is not only about your skincare and the make-up around them but also the eyes themselves.

How can you look after your eyes?

Wear sunglasses to protect your eyes from the sun's UV rays and wear glasses or contact lenses so that you can see properly. You would be surprised to know how many people I meet who go round in a constant blur. It is also important to have regular eye check-ups at your optician's.

Glasses

If you wear glasses, make them part of your wardrobe. Glasses can be an attractive fashion accessory that compliments your personality, colouring and face shape, not something to pretend you aren't wearing. Don't buy a pair that you will only wear in private or that are invisible on your face. You could choose ones that make a statement about your personality, just as your clothes do.

Q How can you choose the best spectacles for your face shape?

(see "Finding your face shape" section)

Firstly, make sure that the spectacles sit correctly on the bridge of your nose. If your nose is long then wear the specs a little lower down and if your nose is short then you can wear them a little higher up. Your eyes must appear to be central in the lenses. If you are very short-sighted or long-sighted, the optical prescription of the lenses may give your eyes a different appearance through the spectacles, so it is important to consult with your optician. But the most important thing is that they feel comfortable and give you good vision. Determine your face shape so that you can choose the best specs. It's all about complementing and balancing your features.

My face shape is oval.
You can wear any shape spectacles. But take your nose shape into consideration and make sure that your spectacle size is in proportion to your face.

My face shape is square.
Never echo your face shape with a square pair of spectacles but wear a softer more rounded or oval shape.

My face is rectangular with a square chin.
You must choose frames which are wide enough for your face shape but which do not echo your rectangular shaped face. But you could wear really strong coloured and sized frames which make a statement on your face.

My face is an inverted triangle shape, with a wide forehead and cheekbones with a small pointy chin.
You should wear frames which are not too wide and do not make your upper face appear wider still.

My face is round.
You should wear frames which are opposite to your face shape, so not round ones. Best for you are square or rectangular shapes that widen your face.

Q *Which colour glasses should you choose*
for your skin colouring?

I have a pinky-toned complexion with fair-hair.
I have a yellow-toned complexion with fair hair.
Both complexion tones will be better with brown, tortoiseshell or lighter coloured frames as you have fair hair. Silver rims are better for pinky-tone skins and gold rims are better for yellow-toned skins.

I am dark skinned.
I have a pale complexion with dark hair.
You can wear strong coloured frames, even black.

I now have white or grey hair
Depending on what shade of grey hair you now have, you can make a fantastic style statement with your glasses. If you used to have black hair with sallow skin that tans easily you could choose a bold, dark or even bright coloured frame. If you were blonde and now you have silvery grey hair then your choice of frame should be lighter coloured, tortoiseshell or silver.

Skincare

There isn't any woman who doesn't look every day and minute of her age. We can't be, nor look, younger than we are, but we can be well preserved.

Lillie Langtry

Your skin is the visual indication of how you have lived your life. Whether or not you are blessed with good genes, if you treat your skin well it will repay you years later by still looking great. If treated with anything less than respect and nurturing, it will be a reminder when you look in the mirror of how constant abuse can destroy a relationship!

Great skin needs you to maintain it in many ways. You can help hold back the ageing process with a healthy lifestyle, exercise, sleep, good nutrition and drinking at least two litres of water a day. Sun exposure, alcohol and cigarettes are all detrimental. Smoking especially can create bad lines around the upper lip.

Careful skincare and minimum exposure to direct sun are the most important things to do to maintain a beautiful complexion. You need to exfoliate, cleanse and moisturise. Toning is less important.

A skincare regime should take no longer than five or ten minutes and once you have a routine it is part of your life. A beauty closet does not need to consist of lots of products, just basic ones that you use twice a day.

Exfoliate

Exfoliation helps to lift dead skin cells and encourage your skin to regenerate before moisturising. Facial exfoliators come in face-washes, wipes, or masks. All will have a similar effect, unless you go to the next level of a mini-peel, which is more invasive and will need to be done professionally.

Cleanse

> *Cleansing is all important. It keeps the skin supple.*
> Julie Andrews

To keep your skin looking its best, you should cleanse first thing in the morning and last thing at night and always remove your make-up before going to sleep (however tired you are). The type of cleanser you use is as much about personal choice as your skin type. Some of you may prefer a cleansing milk; others may prefer oil and yet others may like a foaming wash. Although cleansing pads or wipes are convenient for your overnight bag or holidays, they are not as efficient as proper cleansers. Some of the best cleansers are used together with a hot cloth (soaked in hot water) in conjunction with the creamy wash. The hot cloth will open pores and be more effective in achieving results in your cleansing routine.

Can I just use soap and water?

Never use an ordinary hand soap to wash your face. It will be too drying.

Eye make-up remover

A cleanser may not always do the combined job of face cleanser and an eye make-up remover, especially if removing waterproof makeup, so a dedicated eye make-up remover is necessary.

I never bother to take off my make-up before going to bed.

You must always take off your make-up before going to bed. Otherwise it will soak into your pores and your skin will never get a chance to breathe properly.

When you've finished your cleansing routine, splash your face with cold water. The colder the better; it wakes your skin up and helps circulation. That was a tip from my mother who lived to 91 years old and looked 20 years younger than her age.

Moisturise

When should I moisturise?

Always after cleansing your face first thing in the morning (before applying your make-up),and last thing at night before going to bed. After washing your face, pat in the moisturiser and wait five minutes, if you have time, for it to sink in before applying your make-up.

Should I buy a separate moisturiser for day and night?
Daytime moisturisers tend to be lighter than the night-time ones, which are richer and more nourishing. The more mature your skin, the more nourishing and richer the moisturiser it can take. If you use too rich a moisturiser when you are younger, or have a tendency to an oily skin, you may find your skin becomes clogged and greasy.

How should I apply my moisturiser?
Use a gentle fingertip application with an upward motion so as not to drag the skin downwards. Tap or pat your moisturiser with your fourth fingertips (these exert the least pressure) into the sensitive eye area. Never drag or rub. Skincare is all about treating your skin gently. Massaging your face when moisturising is good for circulation. Increased blood flow will help regenerate skin cells.

I can't afford an expensive moisturiser.
The moisturiser doesn't have to be an expensive brand. Take a tip from the ageless Shakira Caine, Joan Collins or even Yasmin Le Bon who have all used and praised high street brands like Nivea, Olay, Vaseline and E45.

Are there different moisturisers for your skin type?
There is something for everyone. All beauty products, from skincare to make-up, are specially formulated to suit your specific skin type. Some moisturisers will suit your skin better than others, whilst cleansers, toners and make-up removers

are all formulated to work best for your skin type too. Even your foundation can 'work' for your skin (not just its colouring).

In addition to using the correct beauty products for your skin type, it is also important to drink two litres of water daily to hydrate your skin (and body) and eat a healthy diet and exercise regularly.

The types of skin are:

Oily

Your skin is likely to be open-pored and often prone to appearing shiny not long after make-up application. But oily skin usually tans easily and ages better than dry skin, so you are the lucky ones. Mediterranean, sallow skins are usually oily. It is best to use oil-free products on this type of skin, as otherwise they can make an oily skin too greasy and become spotty.

Dry

Dry skins are often pale or freckly Celtic-style skins. Dry skins lap up moisturisers and need lots of care and attention, especially as they age less well than oily skins. Your beauty products should have extra hydrating and moisturising properties.

Combination (usually oily down the 'T-zone' and dry elsewhere)

The T-zone is the forehead, nose and either side of the nose and chin. You can mix and match your beauty products to suit your combination skin. As your skin ages, you may find that your combination skin becomes drier overall.

Mature

Mature skins can be oily or dry but will need richer, more hydrating products to nourish the skin, especially overnight.

Spotty or acne-prone

Even if you have problem skin, you must still moisturise. Using a moisturiser will not create an oilier skin or more spots. If you cleanse and exfoliate regularly and use products specifically for this skin type, you will find your skin can improve. You may also find that a nutritionist's advice on your dietary habits could be more beneficial to your skin than just changing your beauty regime.

Sensitive

Your skin needs gentle products with natural ingredients. Your skin type may be any combination of the above, but needs extra TLC. But extra TLC may mean that less is more in the way of your beauty routine. A simple cleansing and moisturising product may be enough for you with no extra facials, exfoliation or even foundation. You could also find that you are more sensitive to some brands more than others.

Anti-ageing 'super' creams

These creams have all had intensive scientific research behind their development to create a new breed of super wrinkle-busting creams and anti-ageing high performance skin products combining cutting edge bio-technology, pharmaceutical grade ingredients and clinically proven technology.

High street alternatives

If you can't afford the super priced "super" creams, there are many high street alternatives that aim to deliver similar results.

Moisturising serum

A moisturising serum is an extra boost for your skin; you can use it in addition to, and on top of, your moisturiser. You would use it before applying your makeup.

Instant facelift products

As well as serum, there are instant facelift products. These are for use when you look and feel tired and are great to use before a party. A mask can also work wonders to give you an instant glow and lift.

Skin recovery whilst you sleep

Some moisturising products are specially formulated to help your skin recover whilst you sleep. What more could you want?

Eye Cream

Can I use my moisturiser on my eyes as well as my face?

Some moisturisers are too rich around the delicate eye area and may make your eyes puffy. This is why many brands have an eye product to team with the face cream, but the packaging will always have directions for best use.

Multi-purpose skin "healers"

These can be used to help calm or heal dry or irritated skin patches anywhere on the face or body.

UV protection

I know that I must wear a daily sunscreen, so can I buy a combined sunscreen and moisturiser?

Sunburn causes instant ageing, so you should wear a daily sunscreen with at least a factor 15 protection. There are great moisturisers on the market now with this protection included. But to actually sunbathe, I would recommend a dedicated sun tanning product.

Anti-ageing supplements

So you now have a regular skincare routine and can see an improvement in your skin. What else can you do to combat ageing?

You can eat healthily

You need to eat fruit, vegetables and food rich in:

- Amino acids - found in meat.
- Beta carotene (the pigment that converts to vitamin A to help create new cells) – found in sweet potatoes, carrots, apricots, peaches and nectarines.
- Bycopene (helps prevent premature ageing) – found in tomatoes, pink grapefruit and watermelon.
- Omega 3 fatty acids (helps moisturisation of the skin) – found in oily fish, walnuts and flaxseed oil.
- Vitamin C (helps build new collagen) - found in citrus fruits and red berries. In recent medical studies it has been shown that taking 3gm of vitamin C daily as an antioxidant can help combat ageing.
- Selenium – found in fish, red meat, chicken, grains and eggs.
- Vitamin E (antioxidant that combats cell damage and free radicals) – found in nuts, seeds, avocadoes and green vegetables.
- Zinc – mostly found in meat, fish and other animal products; especially high in oysters, crab meat, red meat, chicken and eggs. Medical studies have shown that taking zinc can affect the skin cell structure in a positive way for anti-ageing. You could take a daily zinc tablet, but never on an empty stomach. Doses should be small.
- Folic acid – found in foods that contain folate, the natural form of the acid, including fortified breakfast cereals, dried beans, leafy green vegetables and orange juice.

Medical studies have shown that taking 400mcg daily can help the regeneration of skin cells.

In addition to eating healthily, you can take extra supplements, or combination of supplements, which are specifically for anti-ageing. You can find these at your local health food shop. It is important to consult your doctor before taking any vitamins or supplements.

What else should I do on a regular basis?

- Keep sun tanning on the face to a minimum.
- Keep cleansing, toning and moisturising regularly.
- Drink two litres of water a day.
- Drink less alcohol.
- Don't smoke.
- Sleep on your back. If you sleep on your side or race down, the pressure on your face causes the skin to wrinkle, especially the nasal-labial fold – that is the line down from the nose to the mouth. Laughter lines or crow's feet can also form from sleeping this way, so if you wake up and find yourself on your side or front, turn over onto your back. (Yes, it sounds daft, but I know celebrities who do this!)

Facials

Facials cleanse, tone and moisturise the face. They help the circulation and in bringing fresh blood supplies to the skin can make you look fresher and reduce the appearance of fine lines and wrinkles by temporarily tightening and toning the skin. Salon and spa facials are likely to be more effective than over-the-counter ones for use at home, but all will give you a temporary "feel good" factor.

Mini-peels

A mini peel is more intense than a facial and will help renew your skin cells by exfoliating the surface layer.

Micro-dermabrasion

You could try at-home micro-dermabrasion that will also help to renew and resurface the skin.

What about facial exercises?

Regular facial exercises may prevent or help wrinkles as the facial support muscles support the skin, but could also cause new facial lines to develop during the exercises

Cosmetic acupuncture

If you're looking for an all natural lifting treatment that really does make a difference then you can try cosmetic acupuncture. You will need to have a course of at least six, monthly treatments to really make a difference. But, as with any course of treatments, you will need ongoing monthly treatments to maintain the changes.

Is there anything else new?

In the USA, the search for the holy grail of everlasting youthful looks has turned to a high tech company called

Dermagenetics. This company tests your DNA and formulates a face cream specifically suited to your unique skin cell DNA. They test your cells for collagen breakdown, photo-ageing, wrinkling, skin ageing, and overall health. This test and cream costs around the same as a top of the market luxury brand but it could be quite 'cool' to say that your face cream was matched specially to your DNA – although it has yet to be proved that this new system actually works.

Home anti-ageing mini 'spa' machine

These machines can tone you from top to toe, helping you look younger with healthier skin and a more toned body. The galvanic current helps the body absorb the accompanying products dependant on which part of the body you are treating.

Prescription creams

Retin-A: this is the only proven, effective anti-ageing cream on the market that can dramatically affect how the skin actually looks. It renews the skin cells by allowing new cells to grow after causing old outer layer of skin to be shed. You would use it nightly for a prescribed period of time and then maybe twice weekly, according to how you react to it. It can, though, cause your skin to become sensitive and you must always use a sun protection factor min 15+ afterwards.

Non-surgical procedures

> *The trouble with plastic surgery is that after 10 years, gravity wins out and you have to have another one in a year or so.*
>
> Linda Evans

> *I think people have surgery for psychological reasons more than because of their looks.*
>
> Francesca Annis

> *It is sad to grow old but nice to ripen.*
>
> Lauren Bacall

Although you can never look too thin or too young in Hollywood, there has been a gradual shift away from 'nip/tuck surgery' to just having gentle tweaks without going under the knife. The new message is that it is now cool to be comfortable with your age, with the help of non-surgical procedures giving a subtler, softer look.

The aim is to look naturally beautiful like Kirsten Scott-Thomas.

> *I will never cut my face. I just do a lot of anti-ageing things to slow the process down.*
>
> Eva Longoria

When I am consulted by my clients, I recommend and work

with many of the world's top cosmetic surgeons, skin doctors and beauticians, so I see and hear about all the latest treatments. For the following non-surgical procedure advice I consulted with Bassim Matti FRCS (Fellowship of Royal College of Surgeons) who is a consultant plastic surgeon and the UK secretary of the International Society of Aesthetic Plastic Surgery society (ISAPS), the British Association of Plastic Surgeons (BAPS) and the British Association of Aesthetic Plastic Surgeons (BAAPS).

The non-surgical procedures I have mentioned here are constantly being updated with new products on the market, so I have given an overview, instead of being too specific.

Non-surgical options work best as methods of preventing ageing rather than ways of removing the signs of ageing that already exist. Non-surgical techniques are procedures that do not require surgical incisions or cutting into the skin. The results are mostly immediate; anaesthetic and recovery from the surgery is not required, although some do need skin healing recovery time.

These treatments will *improve* the current you, maybe ironing out a wrinkle or two, filling in a line or smoothing your skin.

As with most beauty treatments they do need maintenance top-ups to be repeated a couple of times a year. The plus side of them is that they are reversible or non-permanent so that if you don't like the effect it's not a catastrophe.

So what are the non-surgical options?

Skin peels

A skin peel renews skin cells by peeling away the very top layer of the skin surface. A peel can improve skin imperfections from acne scarring to fine lines and sun damage.

Are there different sorts of peels?

A mild skin peel contains alpha hydroxy glycolic acid. After a light or mild skin peel you will not need any healing time. Alpha hydroxyl acid (AHA) peels are good at reducing the appearance of fine lines and wrinkles and improving the tone, colour and texture of the skin. You could have a light peel done as often as once a month up to six months and then maintenance peels every two to three months afterwards.

A medium peel is applied in the same way as the mild skin peel. But it can sting briefly when applied. It is good for fine lines and wrinkles and will have a longer lasting impact than the mild peel.

A deep acid peel contains a 20 – 30 per cent glycolic acid and you will be need to be out of action for at least ten days for recovery time as your face will look like it has been burnt. It can improve sun damaged skin, fine lines and wrinkles and mild acne scars.

A laser peel or skin resurface is a much stronger and invasive peel and it takes about a week to heal. It can help age lines, sun damage, skin texture and give your skin a more toned and taut appearance.

Can there be any negative side effects?
You should never use a formula with more than 10 per cent glycolic acid at home as you could end up with facial burns.

A chemical peel gives a smoother, brighter complexion but should not be used too often. The continuous action of artificially creating cell renewal will stop the skin's natural ability to heal itself and produce healthy collagen and elastin.

Scarring is more likely to develop with a medium or deep laser peel or laser resurfacing than any of the mild peels.

A peel can trigger off cold sores if you are prone to them.

You will be more sensitive to the sun. You should try to avoid the sun for at least six months after a major peel.

Peels and laser resurfacing can cause pigmentation problems and may be more successful on fair skinned people than dark.

Laser treatments
Are there are different sorts of laser?
Yes there are. Lasers can be used for hair removal, tattoo removal and the treatment of scarring, acne scarring, fine lines, wrinkles and thread veins, and pigmentation changes.

IPL (intense pulsed light) laser treatment works for fine lines, brown spots and changes of pigmentation, birth marks and scars, tattoo removal, broken capillaries, hair removal and skin rejuvenation. This laser treatment delivers an intense light to a specific area and is gentler and has no recovery time, although you might get some redness immediately afterwards. You will need a series of treatments over weeks. You can see an improvement usually after four to six treatments.

Does laser hurt?
It depends which type of laser treatment is being administered and where on the body is being lasered. Some parts of the body are more sensitive than others. You can have a topical anaesthetic cream applied to help numb the skin. With most laser treatments you will feel a burning sensation, although some surgeries/salons use a cooling device simultaneously to the laser treatment.

How long will it take to heal?
According to the type of laser treatment, recovery can be immediate to around three to five days. If you have had laser on the face you may be advised to not wear make-up straight away and swelling, redness, dryness and flaking are all possible.

What can go wrong?
Skin discolouration and scarring if not used correctly.
After any laser treatment, sun exposure is always best avoided.

New facelift alternatives
Thermage and Polaris treatments use radio waves to

penetrate the skin and heat the collagen under the skin causing the skin to shrink and tighten. This can help give the skin a fresher look after multiple sessions and then maintenance treatments. They can work well on tightening the neck and the results can last up to 18 months.

Injected absorbable non-permanent fillers

Collagen is the best known, proven, non permanent filler that has stood the test of time with rare allergic reactions. It is used most often for the lips. Your body naturally contains collagen, but as you age, the collagen in your skin starts to diminish and fine lines and wrinkles start to form. Injections of collagen work instantly and can last from three to six months.

What are some of the absorbable non-permanent fillers?

Restylane is the most well known of the absorbable non-permanent fillers. These all contain hyaluronic acid which is a non-animal bio-engineered product and a natural substance already present in the body's connective tissues which helps keep the moisture locked in. Hyaluronic acid diminishes in the body There are different versions of filler for separate areas, such as fine lines and deeper wrinkles on the face, the neck and lips.

There are also non-animal derivative fillers that don't contain hyaluronic acid and can last up to six months. These can be best for lips.

Filler injections are commonly used to smooth out face

wrinkles, plump lips, and correct acne scars. They also can reduce lines on the forehead and brow, plump eyebrows or temporal region, fill in under eye hollows, enhance cheek volume and jaw line, soften scars, and reduce aging appearance of hands

Side effects can include swelling, bruising, lumps, and bumps appearing after injection.

How do some celebrities look eternally youthful?
This is the 'pillow cheek' treatment that possibly has been making Madonna and many celebrities look fantastic, but sometimes overly full-cheeked. It adds volume to the upper part of the face by injecting fat right onto the bone, not only eliminating wrinkles (especially the nose-to-mouth lines), but also giving an instant facelift. But it is important to know when to stop as the ultimate goal of a non-cosmetic procedure is an improved you- not a different you!

Are there questions I should I ask?
- What is the filler you are going to use on me derived from?
- Animal, natural or synthetic?
- What are the side effects?
- Could I have a reaction to it?
- Could I be allergic to it?
- What can be done if I am?
- Can it be removed?
- Will I get bruising or swelling after these filler treatments?

You may get minimal swelling, and there is the possibility of bruising as there is with any injection.

Injected semi-permanent fillers
These are usually used for nose to mouth lines.

When injected, they provoke the skin to generate new collagen which fills out hollows and deep wrinkles. The results are gradual over months and require a series of three treatments.

These are all semi-permanent and are generally safe but can cause problems such as lumps. They aren't good for the lips but are better for filling out cheeks and hollows.

Should I choose permanent, semi-permanent or absorbable non-permanent?
Bassim Matti suggests always choosing absorbable non-permanent fillers as they are absorbed gradually by the body and are safer. Semi-permanent and permanent fillers can cause a reaction and are very difficult to remove.
What are the possible side effects?
The side effects of semi-permanent or permanent fillers can be scarring or lumps and bumps. You may need surgery to remove the filler leaving scarring.

Botox
Botox is the most commonly used, non-surgical procedure of all and it really does iron out crow's feet, wrinkles, forehead lines and frown lines between the eyebrows. *But* it looks so much better when used with restraint. It can leave so many

113

women's faces devoid of any expression. As with most things in life, less is always more.

Botox is a muscle relaxing substance that is injected into the facial muscles. It creates temporary paralysis, causing the muscles under the skin to relax and forehead lines, crow's feet, frown lines, smoker's lip fine lines, downward droopy mouth corners, and neck lines to look ironed out.

Even under arm sweating (the Hollywood stars have this done before the Oscars) and sweaty palms can disappear. Botox lasts around three to four months and can take years off your face very quickly; it takes only a couple of days to kick in.

Fat dissolve techniques

These dissolve fat in the area injected into. But these are not yet licensed in the UK as there could be long term side effects that no one yet knows about.

SmartLipo laser: this is less extreme than liposuction and offered as a 'lunch hour' fat removal treatment. A laser probe inserted into the skin heats up and melts the membranes of the fat cells, causing the now liquid fat to be excreted through the natural metabolic process over 12 to 16 weeks. This treatment has passed safety tests and is available in a few countries so far including the UK, but does not yet have approval from the FDA (American Food and Drug Administration) although this is not a legal requirement in the UK for it to be administered.

What questions should I ask my surgeon or practitioner?

- What are your qualifications and training?
- What professional bodies do you belong to?
- How long have you been practising and where?
- What do you recommend for me and why?
- What results can I expect?
- What are the risks?
- What are the negative aspects to this treatment?
- What is the healing and recovery time?
- Is there anything I should avoid doing for the period afterwards?

Teeth

You can instantly improve your facial appearance with a great smile and good teeth.

Do you look after your teeth as well as you do your hair?

Do you...

Have regular dentist check-ups and teeth cleans?

Clean your teeth twice a day?

Change your toothbrush regularly?

Floss daily?

Avoid smoking?

Brush your tongue?

Drink lots of water?

If keeping your teeth healthy and clean is not enough for you, you can also improve their appearance. But even though many of the Hollywood stars have whiter, more even looking teeth than those they started out with, perfection isn't really necessary. Lauren Hutten went through her career as a top model with a gap between her front teeth and Madonna also has a gap. It is always much more interesting to look slightly imperfect. If you would like to improve your teeth, however, even just a little bit, there are many instant options.

I don't like the shape of my teeth.

The dentist can file with a sort of mini electric sander any chipped or uneven teeth or change the size of your teeth with bonding. Bonding is a plastic that can be used to instantly change chipped teeth, re-shape and fill in small gaps. It will last for quite a few years but can chip and discolour with time.

My teeth are crooked.

You can even out your crooked teeth, reshaping them with bonding or veneers.

Veneers are porcelain facades that are created to fit permanently around the front of your own teeth to create a more uniform shape and colour. A tiny bit off the edges of the tooth will need to be filed down to give room for the porcelain veneer. The veneers will give you a brighter, whiter and better smile and can be done within seven to 14 days.

I didn't wear braces when I was a child – is it too late now?
It's never too late! I had my teeth straightened as my 30-something birthday present to myself, wearing braces for a year. In fact I wore clear, fixed braces and no one noticed them even when I was appearing on TV. Eating anything crispy like an apple or a carrot was tricky and kissing was also not too high on the agenda... but I am so much happier with my straight teeth now. Also, it is much easier to floss and brush them to keep them clean and healthy when they are not so crowded.

How about teeth whitening?
Hydrogen peroxide solution is painted on the teeth and subjected to a laser that speeds up the bleaching process. This procedure can lighten the teeth by up to 11 shades. You can get the Hollywood smile like this but it can leave your teeth more sensitive. There are many methods of whitening and 'Zoom' whitening can cause less sensitivity than other whitening methods.

You cannot choose the exact shade of your new tooth whiteness with a laser whitening treatment. It's not a perfect science. So don't believe a dentist when he says you can... Also all teeth whitening will fade again with time. Any bonded or crowned teeth will not become bleached. There are many teeth whitening home kits in the high street chemists that will help make your teeth appear cleaner and brighter which is a good start, but in my opinion its always best to go to your dentist – even if it's a whitening kit you take home from him to use as you will be under proper supervision and teeth can become overly sensitive when bleached.

Can toothpaste help?
There are now all sorts of whitening toothpastes on the market. Some claim to help protect against ageing with vitamin E or folic acid included in the ingredients. Others claim to whiten and can be used occasionally or on a regular basis according to how non-abrasive the ingredients are.

If you brush your teeth and floss regularly, not only will you have a great smile but also nice fresh breath. However good you look and feel, bad breath is a big turn off.

Choosing the right colour for your face

> *The best colour in the whole world is the one that looks good on you.*
>
> Coco Chanel

At times when you become more hormonal, for instance when you reach the menopause, you will find that your skin tone, eye colour and hair colour all change. As you age, your hair may become darker, duller or grey, your skin will be affected by the environment and sun damage, and your eye colour may also change slightly. This is why you shouldn't stick to the same make-up colours, hair colour tints or even the same clothes colours over the years. The colours of the clothes that you wear affect how you look and feel. They can affect your mood, your energy and how others view you. Remember, you only have 30 seconds to create a first impression when you meet someone! So you don't want to look dull or boring or, conversely, too 'over the top'.

Do you wear colours that suit your facial skin tones?

Everyone has skin tones that can be categorised simply as warm (yellow-toned) or cool (pink-toned). Yellow-toned skins tan easily, whilst pink-toned skins usually have difficulty tanning or are freckly. So when you consider your hair colour, your make-up and your clothes, you need to think about your skin tone.

I look tired and drained some days.
Black can drain the colour from your face and make you feel and look tired and older.

If you have to wear black, team it with a colour near your face to compliment your skin tones. You can use jewellery, scarves, shawls, or a glimpse of a t shirt underneath a jacket.

I prefer not to be noticed so I wear beige.
Beige is a non-threatening, safe colour but it is important to try various tones of beige near your face and see which ones

drain your skin colour and which ones lift. A warmer beige will work better on a yellow-toned skin.

I am frightened of wearing colour.
Colour can help you feel and look more youthful. Even if you are scared to wear bright red there is no reason why you can't wear other flattering shades for your specific skin tone, that will lift your spirits, confidence and how you appear to others. But choose your colours with care as some may only need to be worn as an 'accent' colour under a jacket or as an accessory, as the colour could overpower you if too vibrant.

But I like certain colours even if they don't suit me.
But which shade of a colour suits you? For example, you may say you *like* pink but it doesn't seem to suit you. Have you tried putting a pink with blue undertones such as baby pink or fuchsia near your skin, and then trying a pink with yellow undertones such as a coral? One will look much better and 'illuminate' your face. If you have a pink-toned skin the blue-toned pink will look best and if you have a yellow-toned skin then the coral will look best. The same goes for your foundation and lipstick tones.

I don't understand how to choose the right shade.
The correct colour should light up your face. It will make you look fresher and younger. It will bring out the colour of your eyes. It will make people notice *you*, not what you're wearing.

The following is a basic colour guide to help you choose the colours that suit you. You may find that a certain colour, even if you now know the correct shade or tone, may need to be paler or darker to be best for you. It's quite subtle and you will find that all colours are different in daylight than in artificial lighting. That's why you always need to check both your clothes and your make-up in daylight if your lighting in your bathroom or bedroom isn't very good.

Wearing the best colour for you is not an exact science and I would never advocate any woman walking around with their suggested specific colour swatches to clothes shop with. But I do think that from these basic suggestions you can understand why some colours will work better with *your* skin tones than other ones, and avoid making the mistake of buying clothes in colours that don't suit you. (Black is not a mistake, it's just a safe option).

Dark hair with tanned skin, or skin that tans easily

- Best in clear strong colours.
- Celebrity examples: Jennifer Lopez, Halle Berry, Elizabeth Hurley
- Purple, bright red, electric blue, emerald, bright turquoise, fuchsia, yellow, black, white.

Brown or dark brown hair, red hair, fair hair with pale skin, freckles or skin that doesn't tan easily

- Celebrity examples: Nicole Kidman, Julianne Moore, Erin O'Connor.
- Brown, green, gold, khaki, turquoise, charcoal, purple, white.

Fair hair, with golden skin that tans easily

- Best in warm-toned colours with some depth and life in them, rather than cool-toned ones. For example, a warm shade of camel is better than a dull flat shade of camel as this will be draining.
- Celebrity examples: Scarlett Johansson; Kate Winslet, Elle Macpherson.
- Mid-blue, mid-green, yellow-red, turquoise, mid-brown, warm camel, light grey, taupe, coral, cream.

Light 'Nordic' blonde hair, pale skin with pinky tones that doesn't tan easily

- Best in clear, 'cool' pastels.
- Celebrity examples: Grace Kelly, Gwyneth Paltrow.
- Baby pink, baby blue, lilac, pale turquoise, primrose, white, icy grey, eau de nil, maroon, pinky brown.

White or grey hair

- For those who had dark hair and skins that tan easily, best in clear strong colours as in the earlier category. For those with once-blonde hair, best in either of the blonde categories of colour according to the type of blonde you once were.

Accessories for your face shape

Q Do you know what accessories to wear to compliment your face shape?

My face shape is oval.
- Celebrity examples: Scarlett Johansson, Beyonce Knowles, Charlize Theron.
- You can wear any style earrings unless you have a short neck, in which case keep away from long dangly ones.

My face shape is square, with my cheekbones in line with my jaw.
- Celebrity examples: Sarah Jessica Parker, Paris Hilton.
- You can wear earrings that do not echo your facial squareness; softer shapes which hang or rounded shapes such as hoops etc.

My face shape is rectangular with a wide jaw.
- Celebrity examples: Jennifer Aniston, Minnie Driver.
- Do not wear earrings that attract attention to your jaw line. You would be better with studs or small earrings.

My face shape is an inverted triangle with cheekbones and a small pointy chin.

- Celebrity examples: Kate Moss, Cameron Diaz, Jennifer Lopez.
- You can wear any big earrings from hoops to drops that attract attention to, or broaden your jaw line.

My face shape is round.

- Celebrity examples: Gwen Stefani, Christina Aguilera, Renee Zellweger, Kirsten Dunst.
- Do not echo your face shape by wearing hoop or round shaped earrings. It is best to keep to small, understated and subtle, or long and dangly.

Hair

Hair and how you feel are often related. A bad hair day can make you feel unattractive whilst great hair makes you feel positive and good about yourself and therefore more attractive. How your hair is groomed can also influence how you are perceived. Sleek equals 'controlled and professional'. Curly or wavy can indicate sensuality and sexiness and being more relaxed.

Put up hair can make you feel more glamorous and draws attention to the neck and décolleté. Hair colour too can give off signals.

Do blondes have a better time? Are redheads only seen as 'gingers' or as sexy, sultry temptresses?

Apparently red shows individuality, strength and sensuality whilst brunettes are seen to be more serious and sophisticated.

> *When anyone asked what I wanted to be when I grew up,*
> *I'd say 'Blond' because to me that represented beauty.*
>
> Jamie-Lynn Sigler

What is the best hairstyle for your face shape?

Knowing your face shape will help you choose the best hairstyle, make-up and spectacles for you. See the section on determining your face shape – page 64.

My face is round.
Hairstyles that are layered and cut into, taking away the weight of the hair, creating a style that lengthens and frames the face, without making it appear rounder.

My face is long.
Your hairstyle should help shorten the face with a fringe or a cut such as a textured chin length bob.

My face is oval.
Yours is the perfect face shape that suits all hairstyles. However, your age, together with your size (fat or thin) and neck length (short or long) will affect your choice of style. If

you are over 50 then it is probably better not to have one length long hair as it will drag your features down and be more ageing.

My face is square.
Choose a hairstyle that softens the square angles of your features. A layered or soft cut that frames the face will be best for you. Do not have a heavy fringe or short bob.

My face is rectangular
Choose a hairstyle that softens your features as the square shaped face.

My face is triangular (narrower at head)
Choose a hairstyle that broadens the top of your head and slims your jaw.

My face is triangular (narrower at jaw)
You can wear most hairstyles just as the oval face.

My nose is protruding or too large/too long.
Balance your nose with a fringe or a hairstyle that has volume over the forehead. Do not have a centre parting as it will draw attention to your nose. Very flat hair at the back of your head will emphasise your nose when you are seen in profile.

I have a weak chin.
Make sure that your haircut does not stop at a point higher

than your chin, drawing attention to it. A haircut which is soft and framing around the face and jaw line is more flattering.

My ears stick out.
You need a haircut that gives width and volume around your ears. Never wear your hair tucked behind your ears or cut in a short style around your ears. It's all about illusion and tricking the eye.

I have a high forehead.
The best way to disguise a high forehead is with a fringe. It doesn't have to be a heavy fringe: it can be a wispy or layered fringe.

Q Does your hairstyle flatter your body shape?

I'm fatter than I would like to be.
Do not wear your hair in any style that creates extra fullness around your face. Keep to sleek, flattering styles. Less is always more. Not too long, not too big, not too curly. Your hair colour can be broken up with lowlights or highlights around the face.

I'm thinner than I would like to be.
Your hairstyle can help create volume around your face. You could try chunky wedge styles, layered styles around the face, messy 'beach -style' or tousled, big hair.

I've just lost lots of weight.

Long hair can make you look even thinner and drag down your facial features, so a bob or a layered cut would be more flattering.

I have a short neck.

If you have too much hair around your shoulders your neck will look shorter still.

Q How can you look 10 years younger with a new hairstyle?

I haven't changed my hairstyle for years.

As you age, you change. We all do. Your weight may remain the same but you will be carrying it in different places and your face shape will be the same but certain features may become more prominent. And of course there is gravity which is always helping everything go south. So your hairstyle needs to lift your features, and compliment your face shape. What suited you 20 years ago is very unlikely to do the same for you now.

> *My hair had grown completely out of shape and when I looked in the mirror, I felt so depressed. So I started looking at middle-aged women who did have very short hair. That's when I realised I'd go for it.*
>
> Francesca Annis

A hairstyle change is always exciting. It can totally change you. Equally, when you have had a life change it's a good time to change or cut your hair.

My hair is still the same length as it has been for the last 20 years.
Long hair drags your face down and can be ageing. Hair framing your face or a chin length bob will take off 10 years.

I would like to wear my long hair up for a party but it has lots of flyaway short ends.
You can use hairspray to keep it in place, either by spraying straight onto your styled hair or onto your hand and then smoothing over your hair.

My hair has been the same colour for the last 20 years.
Never try to go back to your original hair colour as you age, you may find that a warmer or softer shade is more flattering, especially in the case of red heads.

> *I had a grey hair once. But I reversed it.*
> *I didn't pull it out. I just willed it to go away.*
>
> Salma Hayak
> offering Jennifer Lopez advice on her grey roots.

> *I'm not going to let my hair go grey and*
> *walk around with a shopping trolley.*
>
> Julie Christie

My hair is grey.

Never ever have your hair dyed one flat colour to get rid of the grey. The more extreme the colour, the more washed out you will look and actually older, not younger. Keep your tinted hair colour close to your original colour. If it was dark, don't let it be densely one colour, but add some lowlights. It will be more flattering and younger looking. If it was red or blonde you could add some highlights. This streakiness will also help to make the constant problem of visible regrowth less apparent. If you choose to stop dyeing your hair and go boldly back to being totally grey, I suggest that your haircut is chic and stylish as long grey hair just makes you look older than you really are. It can also be very flattering to have silvery-blonde highlights

> *The thing about doing anything artificial to your hair is that you have to look after it. So you're always vulnerable to the weather and time.*
>
> Francesca Annis

So what are you going to do first to create that new you? A new haircut, or a new body shape?

Many women, when suddenly faced with life on their own after a partnership break-up, cut their hair off, or have a radical re-style. Cutting off your locks is as much to do with being perceived as a 'new you', as cutting ties with your old life. Your choice of hairstyle can define how people will see you. Do you want to be seen as sexy, business-like or feminine?

A bob to be worn perfectly groomed, in the style of Anna

Wintour's, Editor of US *Vogue*, says 'sexy, well groomed, controlled and business-like'. Even *very* short hair can look sexy and feminine, when on the right shaped face with good cheekbones. Sharon Stone and Sienna Miller are celebrities who have looked great with very short hair.

Your hair colour can also change how you feel about yourself and how others see you.

> *I feel more chic when I have really dark hair.*
> Lindsay Lohan

Do you care for your hair properly?

> *Don't over blow-dry your hair, use nylon combs or brushes or over wash it. The natural oils are good for it.*
> Jerry Hall

My hair colour fades so quickly after my visit to the hairdressers. Are there products that would help maintain it better?
There are many high street brands that offer shampoo/conditioners/protection for coloured hair.

I swim every day.
Cover your hair with a protective, leave-in conditioning product and wear a swim hat.

I have lots of hair but it's very fine and flyaway. It needs some more body put into it.

Try a volumising product such as a spray or mousse

I don't know how to blow-dry my hair to create volume.

Towel dry your hair first. Then add some product for volume or extra hold. Don't hold the hairdryer on full heat too close to your hair or for too long, as it dries it out. Turn your head up upside down and brush it whilst drying. It gives volume, You can scrunch your hair as you dry it, if you would like messy, wavy, bed style hair.

I can't blow-dry my hair so that it's sleek.

To get best results, it's important to point the nozzle of the hairdryer down the direction of the hair shaft, smoothing it with the directional hot air flow and with the brush. Aim the hairdryer nozzle very close onto the hair wrapped over the brush. Finish off with cold air. It helps shine and also set.

I blow-dry my hair every day.

If you have to blow-dry your hair each day then I suggest you use the dryer on a low heat setting. You can also apply a heat protective hair product before drying.

A powerful hairdryer will help your hairstyle and cut look its best. The higher the wattage, the stronger the airflow, enabling your hair to be dried quicker with less heat. Most professional hairdryers aren't less than 1800 watts.

It is always best to use a lower heat setting and if your

hairdryer has a nozzle you can direct the heat exactly to where you want it – where you have the hair over the brush.

Hairbrushes

The Rolls Royce of hairbrushes are Mason Pearson, made of natural bristle. But you can also get natural bristle ones on the high street.

I use a hair straightener and hairdryer most days.
You must protect your hair from heat with special products formulated for use with high dryers or straighteners. It is especially important to use these protective products on coloured hair.

The most efficient straightening irons should be hot enough to not require you to run them over your hair more than once, so that you don't overheat and damage the hair.

My hair is curly and difficult to manage. My hair has frizz, not curls.
There are many anti-frizz products to help this problem that condition and protect whilst you are styling the hair. They control and define curls and waves, smooth and calm frizz and flyaway hair and give gloss.

I would like to straighten my hair without using irons every day.
You could go to a hairdresser or try DIY at home with a Permanent Home Straightening Kit: this kit is quick and easy to apply, achieving fantastic glossy and straight hair in less

than two hours. It tames curls, waves and frizz, giving you the feel of a professional treatment that you are doing yourself for less money.

My hair needs some TLC as I have not been treating it well.
Try using an extra special shampoo and always use a conditioner, and you could try a hair mask, a conditioning treatment or a leave-in conditioner.
My hair is in bad condition from a summer in the sun.
Even if you condition your hair every day, you may need a more intensive treatment to help give your hair an extra boost of nourishment.

My hair has lost its shine.
To add gloss you could try using a 'hair gloss' product that creates shine and intensifies colour. These are often sprays to be used after conditioning and drying.

I have dandruff.
There are many high street products to help this problem. You can also use an anti-dandruff shampoo to help speed up the removal of an at home, wash-in, semi-permanent new hair colour when you don't like it.

I am losing my hair.
If you are losing your hair due to trauma or illness there are medical treatments that may help. If you are experiencing hair loss due to hormonal changes- such as post pregnancy,

or menopause then good nutrition is paramount and there are extra vitamins and supplements that also may help.

Q *Does your hairdresser understand you and your hair?*

I always take a picture of the style I would like to show my hairdresser.

If you show your hairdresser a style out of a magazine photographed on a celebrity, the likelihood is that you won't get the look when you next go to wash and dry it yourself, even though the style may have looked good when you left the hairdresser.

When hair is styled on a photo shoot, it is teased and sprayed and fixed to within an inch of its life. You have to consider whether you are a low-maintenance hair woman or are prepared to spend time every day recreating this look. If your hairdresser is worth his salt he will advise you to have a hairstyle that works for your lifestyle, your particular type of hair and also your face shape.

I can't create the same hairstyle at home as my hairdresser does.

You won't be able to re-create the same haircut at home as your hairdresser does if it hasn't been cut to work for *your* type of hair. However technically good the haircut is, it still may not work for you. This can be because your hair may be a different texture or thickness.

Points to remember when visiting the hairdresser:

- Your cut should be one that you can manage yourself at home.
- Never put yourself completely in your hairdresser's hands, giving him carte blanche.
- Never just say 'cut it' – ask how much s/he is going to cut!
- Explain exactly what you would like to achieve from your hairstyle in terms of style, manageability etc.
- Be realistic about your face shape, the sort of hair that you *actually* have (straight or curly, thick, thin or fine) when you ask for your new cut.
- Do not sit with your legs crossed when you have your hair cut. You will finish up with a lopsided cut.
- Wear contact lenses, (if you wear both contacts and glasses), so that you can see what is happening.

I'm not offended by all the dumb blonde jokes, because I know I'm not dumb – and I also know that I'm not blonde.

Dolly Parton

The neck and hands

These are the two parts of the body that age the quickest and that we tend to ignore. Neck skin is thin, with few oil glands so can become quickly dehydrated.

136

$\mathcal{Q}$ *How can you maintain your neck's youthfulness?*

I do use moisturiser.
Even if you use moisturiser, always wear sunscreen (at least factor 15), and don't forget to include your neck when applying it to your face.

I have a really lined and old looking neck.
If a moisturising cream is still not doing enough for you then you can try a non-surgical treatment to help hold back time on your neck skin tone and lines.

Injectable hyaluronic fillers can help plump up the skin on the neck (see "Non-surgical procedures" section) as can Mesotherapy. This is a treatment where a gel with active ingredients including vitamins and amino acids is injected into the skin. It is said to stimulate the cell restructuring of the skin. You will need at least three treatments.

IPL treatments for sun damage pigmentation. They will also help tighten skin. These are done in courses of treatments.

- Glycolic peels will help get rid of fine lines.
- Botox can be injected into the neck lines to relax the neck muscles under these lines and soften and smooth out the wrinkles. You will see a subtle change within days.

- Collagen facials will include the neck area and can help rejuvenate the skin
- Retin-A creams on prescription can also help the neck skin as well as the face.

(See Non-surgical Treatments section for more on treatments for anti-ageing.)

Even if you can improve the appearance of the skin on your neck, remember that you can also dress to flatter your neck and body proportions.

> *Perfume should be worn wherever you want to be kissed.*
>
> Coco Chanel

So what's your neck like?

My neck is too short.
- Wear necklines that are open and deep. This will elongate your neck.
- Don't wear jewellery around your neck as it will shorten it.
- Don't wear collars, and if you do, make sure they are small and always worn open.
- Don't have too much hair surrounding your face and neck.

I have a double chin.

Don't wear necklines that accentuate your chin or stop just short of it, such as a high round neck, as they will only serve to draw attention to your chins. Wide open necks are best for you but you could try to cover and disguise with high necklines such as Chinese style stand-up collars or multi strings of pearls or similar.

But look carefully at yourself and see which looks better. An open neck or covered up? You may find that drawing the eye away from the neck by showing other flesh is more flattering. Make sure, too, that there is not too much hair hanging around your neck and shoulders as too much hair will make your neck appear worse. A good hairstyle, cut to frame the face and not accentuate the chin, would be good.

If you have a large bust as well as a double chin, then you must show some chest flesh so that you don't appear to have a mono-bosom from neck to torso. A high-necked top will not be a good look for you. But if you were to wear a cleverly designed high necked top that showed the décolleté too – the glimpse of flesh would break up the mono-bosom look.

I have a long neck.

You can wear any neckline as long necks are elegant and swan like. You can also wear any hairstyle up or down.

I don't know which neckline suits me the best.

Halterneck
Can be worn by most shapes except those with extreme shaped shoulders, ie: not very narrow or very wide shoulders as the halter will make the very narrow look narrower and the very wide look even wider.

Mandarin
This neckline is simple and good for long necks but not good for double chins or short necks.

Roll neck, turtle neck or polo neck
These necklines are only good for those with long necks and small busts. Never wear high necklines with a large bust. It will make you look larger.

V-neck
This neckline suits most shapes. Widen the 'v' if you have broad shoulders. Lengthen the 'v' if you have a short neck.

Cowl neck
This neckline is good for short necks. It is also good for small busts as it adds extra volume over the bust with the fabric drape.

Slash neck/boat neck
This neckline is open and good for short necks, long necks and to broaden shoulders to balance out a wider hipped body shape.

Sweetheart
This fifties style open neckline is flattering to short necks and big busts.

Frills on the neckline
This is only good for long necks and small busts.

Hands

The signs of ageing are difficult to hide on your hands, so they need to be regularly moisturised and cared for. The skin on your hands is thin and needs extra care and attention. Don't forget about them. It's easy to do so.

Looking after yourself doesn't have to take all day. Even if you don't have time to paint your nails or you don't live a lifestyle that lends itself to painted nails, there is no reason why you can't have clean, tidy, well-manicured hands. Your hands are noticed by everyone, from business colleagues to husbands or partners. There is nothing worse than bitten or dirty nails.

I am the worst culprit for having never looked after my hands over the years. My nails have always been good, but I never used washing-up gloves or hand cream and now it shows. You are never too young to start looking after your hands. The rewards will be there in the shape of smooth skin in later years.

Q *So how can you help your hands look better?*

My hands look older than my face.
You can treat your hands to special treatments and TLC when the skin looks tired, just as you would your face. Your hands will respond by looking fresher and smoother, just as your face does.

My hands have prominent veins and some age spots.
To help remove wrinkles and age spots you could try IPL treatments and Glycolic peels to help plump up skin to disguise prominent veins:

Lipsoculpture or fat transfer. Fat is taken say from your bottom and injected into your hands. This can sometimes make them look lumpy, though.

How quickly can I see a difference with the fillers?
You will need to have at least three treatments to see a change.

Will the treatment hurt?
You may experience bruising.

How long will it last?
Around three to four months.

How can I improve my hands with better care?

Keep your nails clean, and all a similar length. Use a daily moisturiser for your skin and give your nails some TLC once a week in the shape of a manicure, even if it's only a quick tidy up. There are lots of products out there that are luxurious and pampering for the hands. They don't cost a lot as even the high street chemists have linked up with celebrity nail therapists to create special nail care ranges.

What's the best way to do a manicure?

- Using an emery board, file the nails across, gently from underneath, leaving the sides straight. Don't file the sides of the nails inward. You should end up with a gently rounded square shape with the sides not filed away into a slant.
- Massage cuticle softener around the edges of the nail.
- Soak your fingers in warm soapy water.
- Gently push back the cuticle, without cutting it. You can cut the little hang nails away, though.
- Massage a good hand cream into your nails and hands. You could use an exfoliator first.
- Wipe away the moisturiser from the nails before painting.
- Apply a base coat.
- Apply the nail varnish.
- Then apply a top coat.
- Finish off with a quick-dry spray or varnish.

What are my essential manicure tools?
- A wooden orange stick with a chiselled end for cleaning under your nails
- An emery board
- Cuticle softener
- Nail polish remover
- Varnish, base coat, top coat

My nail varnish always chips and peels instantly.
Always use a base coat, and a top coat. Wait at least an hour before you do anything with your hands that may smudge your nails.

I always smudge my nail varnish waiting for it to dry.
You can spray your nails with a quick dry spray and be patient.

My nails never grow to be very long – they break or chip.
Try a fortifying cream that will make the nails shine and look healthy once rubbed in.

Body cellulite

A quick blast of cold water, after a hot shower, does wonders for the skin and circulation.

Shirley Bassey

Q What don't you like about your body?

I have cellulite and fluid retention.
You can have cellulite whether you are thin or fat. Your circulation and a sluggish lymphatic system may create water retention. You can try many treatments to help eliminate them but exercise will help most, together with skin brushing and drinking at least two litres of water daily and a healthy diet. On dry skin, brush your body every day with a natural bristle brush from your feet upwards towards the heart.

- Have weekly massages if you can afford it or massage yourself.
- Stay away from fizzy drinks, caffeine and alcohol as much as possible.
- Exercise to speed up your metabolism. Try to walk or jog at least 40 minutes three times a week.

What spa treatments are there for cellulite?

Endermologie
You are massaged with a roller for at least three treatments a week for a course over a month. Then you maintain with at least one a week. It really works. I have cellulite and this is my preferred and most successful treatment.

Universal contour wrap

You are smeared with a warm mud style solution and then wrapped with sea clay soaked bandages. You do lose inches. This treatment is great for a pre-party instant fix. You can also buy a do-it-yourself version to do at home.

What can I do to help my cellulite with exercise?
The more you move yourself the better. Your circulation will improve. Other options in addition to walking, running, exercise classes and the gym are:

Hypoxi Trainer

A 30-minute, three times weekly cycling session with your lower body encased in a low atmospheric pressure, egg-shaped pod machine. This increases your metabolism and stimulates the breakdown of fat and toxins. You must drink lots of water during and after, follow a balanced nutritional eating plan, and not have alcohol for eight hours before and after the exercise treatment. The cycling treatments target the waist, hips, thighs and bum, and the Vacunaut running machine targets the midriff and tummy area. The Hypoxi trainer does work. I've been trying it for my thighs and knees. Celebrity fans:
Cheryl Cole.

Fit Flops

They help you tone your body as you walk, particularly your buttocks. The soles are angled so as you walk you have to

become more upright and your muscles are used more efficiently. They are those who swear by them, including me, as not only are they comfy but they also look stylish.
Celebrity fan: Nigella Lawson.

Power Plate

A vibrating platform on which you exercise and target body areas by holding lunges and poses for a few minutes at a time. This helps to strengthen, tone, improve fitness and flexibility, and eliminate cellulite. Three sessions a week will make a difference.
Celebrity fan: Madonna.

What anti-cellulite treatment creams are there?
There are many to choose from on the market and these can help the appearance of the skin by smoothing and firming with regular use, combined with diet and exercise. But no treatment will work properly unless committed to regularly over a period of at least six weeks.

Is there anything more I could do?
You can also try a detox diet.

Have you any other suggestions that could help?
Brown legs always look better than pale, so you could use leg-tanning make-up.

Other must have products:

A body brush

Ideally, this should be a long handled, natural bristle brush. You should use it daily on dry skin before showering or bathing. It helps exfoliate and also increase circulation, helping eliminate cellulite.

With exercise you can define your muscles and sculpt your legs, lift your buttocks and help those under-arm bingo wings. Toning and firming will instantly help your body shape and you can try to target specific areas with fat-burning exercises. Although those areas will become more toned and therefore appear slimmer with these exercises, you can't actually choose how and from where your weight will disappear. If you are a pear shape you may lose weight from your face and bust first, but you can flatten your stomach and lift your buttocks. Any aerobic exercise will help raise your metabolism, too, which will help weight loss without diet.

What are my glamour tips? Eating well, but not crazily. I never diet. I drink lots of water and exercise.

Teri Hatcher

Everyone goes through a stage where they are not comfortable in their own skin and you have to learn how to be confident and accept yourself. You want to be sexy and have curves, eat whatever you want, because the more you try not to eat, the more you will eat.

Lindsay Lohan

> *You must ask yourself, do you like what you see? How do you feel? Are you healthy? Life's too short to have an eating disorder! I like fresh baked bread and cheese too much.*
>
> Nicolette Sheridan

Did the slimmer you get lost somewhere amongst the kids' fish fingers and chips?

I have just got divorced and I would like to be slimmer now that I am single again.

Do you feel a bit bruised and battered by the experience? Would you now like to change yourself, but feel unable to do anything about creating a new you? You need to take control, regain your self-esteem and turn back into that sexy woman that you were pre-marriage and/or children. Yes, you may be older, and body parts not quite as new, but it doesn't mean that you can't look your best.

> *Rail thin models might look good on the runway, but it's women with curves and a butt who look good in real life.*
>
> Donatella Versace

> *I've never been on a diet, I'm too greedy! If you're in a competitive profession it's quite nerve-wracking and your nerves need food.*
>
> Francesca Annis

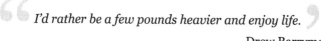

I'd rather be a few pounds heavier and enjoy life.

Drew Barrymore

I will start my exercise regime tomorrow as I have eaten all the wrong things today.

Start your exercise tomorrow by all means, but exercise is not something to do as a penance. It should be part of your daily life. It's important to find a type of exercise that you enjoy doing, otherwise you won't do it. Think positively and if you have eaten all the wrong things today and not done a workout then don't count yourself a failure but just count it a temporary blip and start again on the right path.

I am too old to start exercising now.

You are never too old. But if in doubt, check with your doctor first and be aware of your limitations. If you can afford a trainer or advice, even just once to start you off, it would be fantastic. Or join a health club or your local leisure centre. Look in your library or on the internet for classes. Badger a girlfriend to join you on your daily exercise. Even a short slow walk is a start.

I don't have time to exercise.
- Try to get up an hour earlier.
- Substitute exercise for TV.
- Walk to work instead of driving or taking transport.
- Exercise in your lunch hour.

- Divide your exercise hour into two halves and do one 30-minute session first thing and one before bedtime.

I have never exercised – I don't know how to do it correctly. However you choose to exercise it is important to always warm up and stretch first. Stretching helps your joints to be slowly acclimatised to the movement, to make sure you don't injure yourself and to gradually become more flexible. Warming up is very important; it helps raise your body temperature so that you are less likely to injure yourself and increases the circulation. Since oxygen is carried in the blood to your muscles, the more efficient your circulation the better your muscles will work. It also speeds up your heart rate, ready for you to be even more energetic.

> *Such simple measures as just walking for an hour a day can stop you ending up in a wheelchair or using a walking stick.*
>
> Linda Evans

How often should I exercise?
Everyone should do some exercise daily. Even 10 minutes a day is better than doing nothing at all. For weight loss you should be doing exercise at least three times a week for 40 minutes. The more you do, the more energetic you will feel. Incorporate exercise into your day. Walk up stairs instead of taking the lift. Walk a bit further home from an earlier bus or tube stop, especially if the weather is nice. Try to stand up and

sit down without using your hands to help you. This will strengthen your tummy muscles.

Successful exercising is not about beating yourself up with rigorous routines, but being moderate and consistent. Your choice of exercise has to work for *you*.

Don't give yourself impossible goal posts of exercise regime. Take little steps at a time. Even one step on your journey is better than none.

> *Find the form of exercise that helps you face stress as well as keeping you fit. Swimming can be hugely calming.*
> Shakira Caine

Should I eat before I exercise?
You need energy before you exercise. You cannot have any energy with an empty tum. If you are exercising first thing in the morning, how about trying a fruit smoothie or blend some fresh fruits with yoghurt, or even just a banana?

When I get depressed I can hardly motivate myself to get out of bed, let alone do any exercise.
To help combat depression without medication, it has been shown that going out and doing some exercise – even a brisk walk – can help produce serotonin or 'happy' chemicals in the brain and make you feel happier and more motivated.

I have to spend at least three hours exercising each day otherwise I will be fat again.

If you have had an eating disorder such as bulimia or anorexia and can only control it by over-exercising to compensate for eating, then you need to try to gradually wean yourself off those extreme hours to no more than an hour a day. Try making yourself a chart with reduced hours. Exercise to this schedule and you will see that reasonable amounts of exercise will be as effective too.

I'm embarrassed to go to the gym as I am too fat.

Avoid going to the latest 'cool' gym or classes where you may find that you compare yourself to super fit women who have nothing else to do with their day but workout and look after themselves. Find a course of classes specifically geared to a long term weight loss programme. You will find that there are others like you and it will give you motivation.

I can't run as I have knee joint problems.

It can be just as beneficial to walk. Power walk or walk fast – don't stroll. It's about the energy you put into your exercise. Suitable trainers are very important when you have existing injuries. Make sure you stretch at the end of your walk.

I have a bad back.

Posture is very important. If you have a bad back it is very important to support the back itself with the surrounding muscles. So the more you can strengthen tummy muscles and back muscles the better. When you are exercising, stop before you feel any pain and never do any movements or exercises in a group class that hurt your back. Only do what works for you, not because everyone else is doing it. I've found that Pilates classes are the key to helping improve a bad back as the exercises help strengthen the core muscles that support the back.

If I starve myself for a few days I'll lose weight faster.
Eat regularly and moderately through the day, maybe five small meals. This can regulate your metabolism and keep it burning the calories. When you starve yourself by not eating, your metabolism will stop working as efficiently and you will gain weight, not lose it.

I'll start my diet tomorrow.
Don't make excuses. Tomorrow never comes. Today is the first day of the new you, not tomorrow.

> *A minimum of 50 sit-ups three times a week will give you a well toned stomach and one that you will be able to reclaim quickly even after childbirth.*
>
> Jerry Hall

I am on a constant on–off diet.
The more you yo-yo with your dietary habits, the more you will confuse your metabolism and it will become more sluggish and you will have even less energy. In fact you will become fatter eventually, not thinner.

I get impatient when I diet as I don't lose weight immediately so I give up.

Your current body shape and weight is the result of many months or even years of being that way, so don't give up. It needs time to change slowly and re-adapt to your new healthy living and eating patterns. This will not be overnight or even after a week. It may be a few months before you really start to see a difference.

Do *not* weigh yourself more than once a week. It's all about your body shape and how you look in your clothes, not your weight as muscle is heavier than fat.

> *Your body is the direct result of what you eat*
> *as well as what you don't eat.*
>
> Gloria Swanson

I don't know how to eat healthily.

What you eat affects the whole of you. What you put into your body is like putting fuel into your car. If you run low on petrol your car doesn't run at all, or if you put the wrong sort of petrol in it doesn't run very well. If you overeat it will be stored as fat. When you exercise you will help burn up the fuel that you fed your body with.

You need carbohydrates, good fats, protein, green vegetables and specific minerals and vitamins (through the food you eat or as a supplement). Ideally you should eat a big breakfast, a smaller lunch and an even smaller dinner, keeping all the carbohydrate consumption up to lunchtime.

I eat chocolate and sugary foods to give me energy bursts.
These foods only give you a quick fix energy burst, so that you will have a burst of energy and then slump again. The less sugar you eat, the less you will crave it. To keep you on an even keel, you need to eat foods that are slow energy-release which give you long term energy rather than a quick fix. Good carbohydrate snacks include a slice of wholemeal bread, pasta, sweet potatoes, baked potatoes. A piece of dark organic chocolate would be better than ordinary chocolate. If you are really tired why don't you try a taking power nap for 20 minutes? Eating a small handful of non-salted nuts such as almonds together with a fresh fruit snack will also help an energy surge and slump.

Slow energy-release foods include:
Grainy brown bread (multi-grain, seeded and granary), bran based breakfast cereals, porridge and sugar-reduced muesli, sweet potatoes and boiled new potatoes, pasta with tomato-based sauces, basmati rice and brown basmati rice, grains (bulgur wheat, couscous and quinoa), nuts (no more than a handful a day), fruits (fresh or canned in juice or dried), vegetables (raw, lightly cooked, canned or frozen, though fresh are obviously better), and salad.

Also, you may find it beneficial to eat more often, eating five small meals at breakfast, mid-morning, lunch, tea, and supper. Keep away from all sugary snacks and refined and processed white flour foods such as sugar-rich breakfast cereals, bread, pizza, pies, cakes, sweet biscuits, doughnuts, croissants and sweets.

> *Once you take your first steps on the long journey back to health, there's really no going back.*
>
> Lorna Luft

What are the best foods to eat?

- Beef, lamb, chicken and eggs in moderation.
- Fish and shellfish, but especially oily fish such as salmon, sardines, tuna, mackerel.
- Dairy including milk, low fat cheeses, yoghurts (cow, sheep and goat).
- Soya products
- Seeds and legumes.
- Nuts (not dry roasted but plain, preferably non-salted).
- Potatoes, sweet potatoes.
- Green leafy vegetables.
- Salad (lettuce, cucumber, tomatoes, avocadoes, peppers, cress etc).
- Fresh fruit.
- Porridge.

Keep to grilling, roasting, boiling or cooking with a little olive oil in a pan.

What are the worst foods?

- White flour, cakes and biscuits and anything sugary.
- Chocolate (except dark organic).
- Processed salty foods such as sausages, ham, bacon.
- Pre-packaged ready meals, including low sugar/low fat

labelled ready meals (because they are mostly overfull of salt and other 'hidden' additives to make them tastier).

- Anything fried.
- Anything with too much salt.
- Fizzy drinks.
- Coffee.
- Pizza.
- Hamburgers (unless they're homemade)
- Never eat carbohydrate-heavy meal combinations, such as chips with pasta, pizza and chips, or chip butties.
- Mayonnaise laden salads such as coleslaw, potato salad. Sauces such as ketchup, mayonnaise.

> *Moderation in all things is the key.*
> Joanna Lumley

I keep picking at the wrong things and cheating.
Don't buy these foods for the home. When you shop, make sure that your nibbles are all healthy ones like crunchy vegetables, fruit or even hummus and crispbread, rather than crisps and chocolate. Never do a food shop when you're hungry.

I keep going out to parties and breaking my diet with the canapés.
Eat something proper before you go out, even if you think you might go out to dinner after the party. If you are likely to eat very late, maybe have only a light starter dish at the

restaurant and have your 'main course' at home before the party. That way you won't want to pick. Your dress may feel tighter before you go out, but it won't be even tighter the next day.

So why do you eat?

I am unhappy or depressed.
You shouldn't comfort eat. Food to help your feelings will only make you feel worse when the sugar 'happy' rush has worn off, as you will regret your binge. Food does not make you feel better. You are the only one who can make you feel better.

I am tired and need the food to give me energy.
In the same way that the comfort eating will give you a 'happy' rush, it will also give you instant energy, but energy that isn't long lasting will make you more tired when it ends.

I'm fat anyway – what difference will one more day make.
A day will make *all* the difference. If you start today, tomorrow will already be day two on the way to the new you.

I've given up smoking.
You should eat at designated mealtimes, whether it is three or five times a day. Take the time to actually sit down and chew, savour and digest your food so your brain and body actually register it was a meal, not a snack. Once you've eaten, stop

when you're full, don't have seconds and get up and move away from anywhere food related. If you are in a restaurant finish your meal with a herbal tea, not a calorie laden cappuccino.

I am bored.
Don't use food as a diversion tactic to stop doing whatever you don't want to do and don't use food to cheer yourself up – go and do something else for *you* instead.

Because I'm cooking for and feeding the children.
If you are surrounded perpetually by your kids' leftover food or anything leftover you think you might be tempted by, either freeze it straight away into little containers for future usage or chuck it.

I can't lose the weight from my now menopausal midriff.
This is the most difficult part of the body to shift weight from and the area that most women over 40 dislike about themselves. It is difficult to target a specific area of the body to lose weight from but with general weight loss you should find that there is a slight improvement at your midriff. But you can really help tone up an area by concentrating on it with dedicated exercises. And of course there is clever dressing, which we will come to later.

Menopause

The really frightening thing about middle age is the knowledge that you'll grow out of it.

Doris Day

After thirty, a body has a mind of its own.

Bette Midler

I first started my advocacy for women's health in the field of reproductive freedom, and the next stage would be bringing menopause out of the closet.

Cybil Shepherd

This book is not a health manual or health and beauty directory. So with health related subjects like the menopause, I am going to focus more on how to look good than how to deal with the medical aspects.

When you reach the menopause you may experience a slower metabolism, weight gain, loss of skin elasticity, lack of energy, thinning of hair and a duller complexion and sleep disruption. And your weight is most likely to end up around your mid-body and arms.

So I am going to offer some solutions for dietary additions that may help you through your menopause, but you should always seek professional help from your doctor or nutritionist too.

You could always try an alternative and see if it works for you.

> *I have tried taking Dong quai for menopause*
> *and a plant gel called Estrogel.*
>
> Shakira Caine

Q *What foods and supplements can help you through the menopause?*

I don't want to take hormone replacement therapy.

There are many opinions on the pros and cons of taking hormone replacement therapy (HRT), from doubts about its long-term effects to how wonderful and rejuvenated many women feel when they do take it. There are also natural HRT alternatives. 'Natural' can mean natural as opposed to 'synthetic' hormone replacement and 'natural' as in natural diet and food supplements.

'Anti-ageing clinics' can help you feel good with anti-ageing, non-surgical treatments (see section on anti-ageing) and anti-ageing hormone balancing.

What foods and supplements might be beneficial at this time in my life?

Plant oestrogen rich food

These include

- whole grains (oats, corn, barley, millet, buckwheat, wild rice, brown rice, whole wheat), soya flour and flax seed oil.
- Vegetables, especially green leafy ones.

Herbal tablets

Agnus Castus, Dong Quai, Black Cohosh, Dong Kwai

Nutritional supplements

- Evening primrose oil
- Essential fatty acids – omega 3 and 6
- Folic acid
- Chromium
- Multi-vitamins
- Vitamin B complex
- Antioxidants (vitamins A, C and E, selenium, zinc, magnesium)
- A herbal sleeping remedy

My skin is so dry

Rehydrate your whole body by drinking at least 2 litres of water a day and a richer facial moisturiser specifically created for the mature skin may help too. This does not have to be expensive. High street, inexpensive brands are often just as effective and contain the same ingredients.

Rose and frankincense are two essential oils that are excellent for dry, mature skins. Some moisturisers contain these ingredients or you can buy them as essential oils, a few drops of which you would mix with a carrier oil.

I can't sleep.

You could try a hot bath with a few drops of lavender essential oil added to promote relaxation. Have a hot drink, but not one that has caffeine: a herbal tea such as camomile or a hot milky drink with warm milk. Remove the TV from your bedroom, and try reading a book instead. There are meditation and relaxation techniques and also herbal remedies from your local health food shop that may help promote a more restful night.

> *Eat well and sleep well. That will feed your nervous system and your pysche. As you get older, you look how you feel.*
>
> Francesca Annis

I look old suddenly
A major trauma or serious illness will make you look older, but only temporarily until you recover your state of health and mind again. Don't look in the mirror on a daily basis and think how old you look. If you feel young you will exude youthfulness in your thoughts, speech and actions. NB. I am not suggesting dressing like the proverbial mutton.

Underwear

Whatever your size or shape or weight, good fitting underwear is all important.

Good underwear together with good posture can make a difference to how your clothes look on you.

> *I dress for women, and undress for men.*
> Angie Dickinson

Underwear can make you feel sexier and more feminine or just more confident if it is supporting you properly. Corsetry style underwear can create body shaping solutions underneath difficult dresses, whilst sexy, revealing lingerie together with subtle lighting in the bedroom can do wonders to help you feel sexier and your body look its best.

> *Brevity is the soul of lingerie.*
> Dorothy Parker

Having dressed so many celebrities for the red carpet over the years, I saw how difficult it was to find body shaping underwear that worked under red carpet dresses, and created my own online lingerie shop, www.redcarpetundies.com, for women to buy underwear solutions to re-shape, slim and support.

> *I always wear a matching set, a nice thong and a nice bra.*
> Cheryl Cole

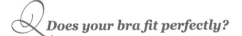

Does your bra fit perfectly?

I haven't been measured since my 20s. I just guess my size now.

When shopping for your new bra, you should make sure that

165

your breasts sit comfortably in the cups, not overhang the cups creating two extra bosoms. The underwire should not cut in and the straps should not dig into the shoulders. You may need a bigger cup size and a smaller back size for a perfect fit.

The majority of women wear bras that are the wrong size. As you age, your body shape changes. So you will need to make sure that your bra size and fit changes with your body shape. Ideally you should be re- measured/fitted every six months.

Where do I go for my bra to be fitted?

The best way to get a bra that fits well is to be measured by an in-store bra fitting expert. But you must find yourself a really experienced fitter as even they could get your sizing incorrect. It is not an exact science. Even if you think you know your correct size, each manufacturer will have a different interpretation of fit and cut. Department stores such as John Lewis and Debenhams have trained fitters who can advise you, as do Rigby and Peller, who have the Royal Warrant. I have been known to go through many of my clients' lingerie drawers and not find one bra there that fits correctly. One of my clients was wearing a bra four back sizes too large and four cup sizes too small.

My bra felt right when I bought it but I'm not sure any more.

Most high street bras have machine washing instructions and have been tested to be machine washed, but no bra will last as well being machine washed, as it will being hand-washed. So you will need to replace your bra more often than you think for it to continue giving a perfect fit. When you buy your bra, fasten it on the loosest hook and then gradually start fastening it on the tighter one as the bra gives and stretches after washing and wearing.

I would like more cleavage.
There are many bras now on the market that have either extra foam padding, or silicone or gel inserts. You can always add extra silicone 'chicken fillet' style inserts for even more cleavage.

My cup size is a DD.
If your breasts are big, it is likely that the best bra for you will have wider straps for support so as not to cut into your shoulders. A good, daily wear bra should hold your bosoms comfortably in place without any overspill. Therefore you may find that a higher, less plunging style cup fits you best. If you want cleavage for evening wear, the best fitting bras for bigger girls will have an extra panel in the outer underside of the cup to give a firmer hold and help push the bosoms together. Good fitting bras are all about the technology and infrastructure, not just their appearance.

I have had a mastectomy, but not yet had a reconstruction.
Having worked with ladies who have had breast cancer, I know that one of the psychological effects of the illness is

feeling a loss of femininity with the loss of a breast or breasts. But it's now possible to find sexy mastectomy bras and swimwear that have special prosthesis pockets. I don't see why these bras should only be functional and not look pretty. It's important for you to feel and look sexy again.

Q *How can you avoid visible pantie line?*

I don't want to wear a thong.
Buy your panties at least a size or two larger than your actual size. Even if you hate accepting that you bought such a large size (cut the label out straight away) you will have less visible lines. Other styles that are best for this are 'boy short' style panties and French knickers. Brazilian style panties are half way between a thong and a pantie with a half-brief at the back.

> *I don't wear stays. What's the point? If you squeeze it in at one point, it only comes out at the other.*
> Lillie Langtry

Don't 'hold-in' pants make the flesh go elsewhere?
If you buy the correct size then there should be no overspill of flesh. Styles that are high-waisted can help too.

I have no bottom, although I am quite a curvaceous, larger woman.

'Contour pants' make your bottom more curvaceous like Jennifer Lopez's. They are panties with foam inserts in the two cheek areas that give a naturally shaped curve. You could even wear the pants under your swimsuit if you are that self-conscious about your flat bottom.

Fashion and style

Even if your public image is all about 'glamour' it doesn't mean that's how you dress at home.

Everyone thinks I'm glamorous, which makes me laugh because I'm pretty geeky. On Saturday mornings I love watching cartoons in my Care Bear slippers and pyjamas set. How's that for glamour?

Mischa Barton

Being stylish doesn't mean dressing up at all times.

Fashion is a part of my work. I feel a responsibility to be presentable, to dress up if the occasion calls for it. But really, fashion does not play that big a role in my life these days. The better part of my day is spent in practical clothing.

Sarah Jessica Parker

Nor does it mean wearing a 'too carefully considered' head to toe combination of current season (or even next season's) brand new designer labels. To me, stylish means throwing together any combination of clothes (new and old) and still looking great, whatever the outfit or occasion. An example would be Kate Moss or Alexa Chung looking as stylish at the Glastonbury pop festival as they do at a black tie gala event. They stand out from the crowd in their choice and mix of clothes and how they wear them with attitude and confidence. But you don't have to be youthful to be stylish; there are so many 50+ women who look stylish. My auntie who is now 89 always looks glamorous and stylish on a shoestring budget.

> *As a teenager, I was forever dressing in black bin liners and anything I'd bought from a jumble sale. I'm not sure that look was entirely successful, but I adored it.*
> Kristin Scott Thomas

Stylish women look relaxed, happy and comfortable in both their own skin and clothes. Older women should be well-groomed and well-maintained, but never look stiff, whilst younger women can be more adventurous. Clothes can affect your mood, so anything that makes you feel and look fatter, shorter, dumpier, frumpier or older should be removed from your wardrobe. Style is not just about what you wear but how you wear it and how you put it all together. It could be a single accessory that makes all the difference to a simple outfit.

> *On the whole, I think women wear too much and are too fussy. You can't see the person for all the clutter.*
>
> Julie Andrews

> *The key to looking good is inner happiness, calm and confidence.*
>
> Fiona Fullerton

Whatever your size, thin or fat, your body shape is going to determine what you should wear. You should not be unrealistic.

> *I love fashion. I love when people put me in it. And God knows, I'm slowly getting better at putting stuff together myself.*
>
> Jennifer Aniston

So who is your style icon?

Who do you admire?

When you dress up, do you dress with her in mind? For example, would you love to dress to be understated like Audrey Hepburn or Grace Kelly? Or do you prefer being more of a trendsetter, like Madonna? Or are you happy just to be you and dress in a style that simply suits you?

> *I am not a trendy person, though I like clothes as much as the average woman.*
>
> Julie Andrews

So who are *you* and do you have a wardrobe that works for all your life? As a mum on the school run? As a working woman during the day? As glamorous wife/lover at night?

Dressing well is a perfectly achievable goal. You should not keep clothes in your day to day wardrobe that are pre-baby (if your children are now grown up), from your pregnancy, from a previous weight loss or gain, or from your last office job that you no longer work in. Even if you own a *classic* little black dress it doesn't mean that it actually still suits you, or that it still looks OK. Your shape may have changed over the years, together with fashion shapes.

In part one, you considered how you feel about your body shape and learned to focus on the positive, not just the things that you would like to change.

Now you are going to dress cleverly to give the illusion of a more proportional body shape, whatever your size.

Ideally, your shoulders should be roughly in line with your hips (if you were to draw a vertical line from your shoulder to hip).

Your bust should be in the right place and with a good shape (big or small – it doesn't matter).

You should have a waist of some sort, even if it's only the space created between your correctly supported bust and your tummy.

There's nothing wrong with womanly curves such as a softly curved tummy and a proper bottom. Most men prefer women with curves.

Legs should appear to be as long and slim as possible.

> *I laugh when I end up on the worst-dressed list. I'm not trying to be fashionable. I know I'm kind of a cartoon character. Do people honestly think I'm wearing a kaftan in order to be fashionable?*
>
> Pamela Anderson

My style tips:

- Less is always more; go for an understated look.
- Understand your body shape and dress for it.
- Be honest with yourself about your size and buy the right one. If it's not the size you want to be, cut the label out.
- You have to be comfortable in your own skin to be comfortable in your clothes.
- Never show cleavage and leg together. One or the other.
- If you wear a baggy top, team it with a slim fitting bottom.
- If you wear a tight top, team it with a looser fitting bottom.
- Buy clothes to wear that you are comfortable in now, not those that will fit you when you may be thinner next week.

> *It is the unseen, unforgettable, ultimate accessory of fashion that heralds your arrival and prolongs your departure.*
>
> Coco Chanel

> *[Style] is an expression of individualism mixed with charisma. Fashion is something that comes after style.*
>
> John Fairchild

It's about your simplicity. Showing your eyes. Making your dress disappear. It's not pushing it too much – it's all about you.

Alber Elbaz, designer

> *Fashion is what you adopt when you don't know who you are.*
>
> Quentin Crisp

How can you change your body shape with clothes?

You can use specific clothes to create an illusion to balance and flatter. You can use colour, cut, and specific style rules to suit and enhance your own body shape.

Using colour for your body shape, mood and first impressions

> *The best colour in the world is the one that looks good on you.*
>
> Coco Chanel

Your body shape will look its best when you consider what colours you need to wear to attract the eye to your best bits and distract from your worst bits. Colour can also make a difference to how you look and feel, and how others see you.

If you would like to play safe with the colour palette in your wardrobe then the key classic colours are black, white, camel, cream, grey, navy blue, brown.

If you create a wardrobe around these basic colours then you will need to add some brighter colours or patterns to give life, light and shade to your outfit. These are called accent colours.

Just remember I like terribly simple clothes and I hate prints.
Jacqueline Kennedy
writing to her fashion advisor in 1960

Always be more important than your clothes.
Paris Hilton

You can always play safe with a little black dress, but other colours can be slimming too, such as dark grey, chocolate brown, maroon and navy. Darker colours will help distract the eye whilst lighter ones will attract the eye.

In the same way as lighter or brighter colours, shiny fabrics and large or busy prints will also attract the eye. Think which part of the body you would like to look slimmer and wear the darker plainer colour on that part of you.

How shall I wear prints?

If you are a curvaceous plus-sized lady, with a big personality you can get away with a big print, but a print on a darker background may be more flattering.

Q *Can you define your body shape?*

The following is a simple guide to body shapes. I have given celebrity examples wherever possible to help you visualise the shape I am describing, but obviously this isn't an exact science; everyone's body is different and there will be variations within each body shape. Be honest with yourself and try to work out which body shape best describes you, then take this as a starting point for your fashion decisions.

Are you a voluptuous but slim hourglass?

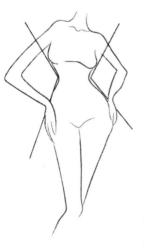

I wear the same size top and bottom. I am slim but curvy with a defined waist and bust and bottom. I want to show off my curves and define my waist.

Celebrity examples: Halle Berry, Liz Hurley.

I feel that everyone talks to my bust when they talk to me.

Celebrity examples: Kelly Brook, Jane Ross (Jonathon Ross' wife). You are so lucky to have those curves. Most women would love to have a curvaceous shape.

You put on an outfit and you think "Hey I look sexy". But I think it's rare that you feel beautiful. I think beauty is something that you sort of recognize in other people. I never look at myself in the mirror and say, "I look really beautiful".

Scarlett Johansson

Best shapes for a voluptuous but slim hourglass:

The best styles for you are those that accentuate your fabulous figure. Decide how much cleavage you wish to expose, but balance it with less leg on show, however good your legs are. Less is always more, even if you have the perfect body.

Are you a curvaceous, fuller-figured hourglass?

I have a large bust and hips and if I buy clothes to fit my bust and hips, the waist is always too big.

Celebrity examples: Nigella Lawson and Helen Mirren.

Best shapes for a curvaceous fuller-figured hourglass

It is very important to have your bust correctly supported, to create as much space as possible between bust and waist to show off that hourglass figure and that you really do have a waist.

Simple shapes with no frills or flounces will be more flattering; V, wide and slash neck tops and wrap dresses will create a less busty look. Avoid shapeless styles that fall from the bust. Mono-block colour dressing can help to create a slimmer silhouette.

Are you a triangle or pear shape?

I wear a larger size on my bottom half than my top half and if I put on weight I carry it on my hips and thighs.
Celebrity examples: Sharon Osbourne, Oprah Winfrey.

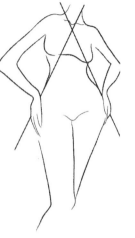

I am slim but my hips and bum are bigger than my top half.
Celebrity examples: Gwyneth Paltrow, Jennifer Lopez,

Best shapes for a triangle or pear shape

Necklines that broaden your shoulders to balance out your hips include wide V-shaped, slash-necked and off the shoulder, whilst layering such as a jacket over a shirt over a T-shirt will take the attention away from the hips. The layers can end at various lengths. You could even layer a knee length dress over floppy trousers.

One-shoulder styles or styles that give an asymmetrical illusion are very flattering.

Lighter, brighter colours or patterns worn on top and dark, plain colours on your bottom half will create an illusion of balanced body shape. Avoid halter necks, which draw the eye inwards, and sleeve shapes that can narrow the shoulders

Keep any volume to your upper torso; never wear skirts or trousers with pleats or gathers.

Are you an inverted triangle?

I am slim with broader shoulders than hips and a good bust, but no defined waist.

Celebrity examples: Anna Kournikova, Sharon Davies.

I have wide shoulders, and no waist or hips.

Best shapes for an inverted triangle

Simple, non-fussy styles that create volume over the hips to balance out the width of the shoulders. Distract the eye from the larger top half with a darker colour top teamed with a lighter coloured bottom.

Are you are a lean column?

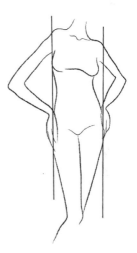

I wear the same size top as bottom, have a small bust, a small but non-defined waist and definitely no hips. From the front I look straight up and down, but if I put on weight I do have a bottom.

Celebrity examples: Cat Deeley, Nicole Kidman.

I have a boyish shape although I do have a bust.

Celebrity example: Uma Thurman.

Best shapes for a lean column

Create curves and volume using detailing and cut, such as ruffles, gathers or stitching

Shifts, columns and asymmetrical, one-shouldered dress shapes will flatter. Colour blocking (contrasting blocks of colour) can break up your lean column shape).

Are you an apple or a rectangular body shape?

I carry all my weight around my middle and have no waist now. However slim I get, I still have flesh around my midriff, but I do have good legs.

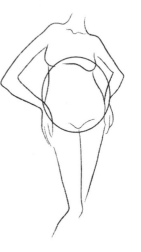

Celebrity examples: Joan Collins, Cilla Black, Judy Finnegan.

Best shapes for an apple or rectangle

Simple styles in soft fabrics which drape and skim or wrap over the curvier areas.

Wide, V or slash necklines will help create a balanced body shape.

Are you petite?

I am only just over five feet tall.

Celebrity examples: Reese Witherspoon, Lucy Liu, Kylie Minogue, Sharon Osbourne

Whether you are a beanpole, curvy, pear-shaped, big-busted or plus sized, if you are petite you *must* dress to suit your proportions as well as your body shape. You will need to consider things like your arm length, body length, and whether you have a short waist or short legs. Try to always buy from petite ranges as the proportions will be correct for you. You will find that sleeve lengths are better and the waists are in the right place.

Best shapes for petite
You are best in one colour from head to toe to give the appearance of height.

Petite body shapes look best in simple clean shapes that skim the body.

Everything should be proportional, so accessorise with small accessories.

Extra long jeans over high heels can add the illusion of height as can nude coloured shoes to elongate the leg.

Do you dress to flatter your bust size?

"*What's so beautiful about breasts is their uniqueness. I don't understand the obsession with fakeness. It's a very odd thing, isn't it, to prefer fake and big to small and unique or just beautiful and real.*"

Anne Heche

I have a large bust.
Celebrity examples: Salma Hayek, Scarlett Johansson, Drew Barrymore.

> *There's something very awkward about women and their breasts because men look at them so much. Men love them, and I love that.*
>
> Drew Barrymore

Best shapes for a large bust
Flatter a large bust with wide open necklines, wrap dresses and most importantly well-fitting bras. A proper bra can change your body shape and give the illusion of dropping dress sizes instantly. Never wear frills or detailing on the bust line or styles that fall from the bust. Make sure that there is space under your bust at your midriff. This will accentuate your great figure shape.

> *I love my boobs. My sister Jessica grew up having a larger chest. Men love it and stare at it, but she needs to wear two sports bras to even play volleyball. My point is that whether you have big boobs or small boobs, there are always pros and cons.*
>
> Ashlee Simpson

I have a small bust.
Celebrity examples: Gwyneth Paltrow, Calista Flockhart, Kate Moss, Paris Hilton.

You can wear most styles. Small busts do have some advantages.

> *I like being flat. I think it's hot. I never have to wear a bra. When I was 13, I really wanted a boob job because all my friends started to have boobs and I was the only one who looked like a boy.*
>
> Paris Hilton

Best shapes for a small bust
If you wish to add the appearance of volume over your bust area, add detailing such as pockets, buttons, frills, gathers, ruching, beading and patterns.

Padded bras and silicone inserts can give extra cleavage.

You can wear plunging, barely there dresses without worrying that everything is hanging out and without the need for a bra to hold everything up. You are very lucky.

I'm a fuller-figured girl.
Celebrity examples: Queen Latifah, Vanessa Feltz;
You can show off your cleavage and even your curvaceous bottom with pride, in clothes that flatter. Big women are sexy.

Best shapes for the fuller figure
Styles that gently skim your shape. You still want to show you have a figure.

Simple, non-frilly wrap over and low V-neck styles work best for your body shape.

If you wear an outfit that you feel is too close fitting, try a sheer, looser layer over the outfit to disguise subtly but not hide completely.

You may prefer to always cover your upper arms.

Do clothes never fit at your waist?
I am short-waisted.

Create an illusion to cheat the eye into thinking that your body is longer than it is.

Define the area between your bust and waist by wearing a well fitting bra.

Wear your tops layered to create a longer body length and never a wide belt.

One colour on top and bottom will help lengthen the torso.

I am long-waisted.

You need to cheat the eye into thinking that your body is shorter than it is, by bringing the waistline up. So you can break up your silhouette with blocks of colour. Empire line or high-waisted styles will also create the illusion of a shorter body.

What are your arms like?
I have short arms.

Make sure that your clothes, especially your coats and jackets, have the correct length sleeves. When your sleeves are too long, you can look as though you are wearing someone else's clothing. Three quarter length sleeves can be very flattering for you.

I have flabby under-arm bingo wings.

You can cover with shawls, shrugs, wraps, boleros or anything sheer, lace or sequinned that conceals and detracts the eye without hiding your arms completely.

Do you have a tum?

I hate my tummy.

Flat-fronted skirts or trousers without pleats or gathers are your best friend..

You can distract with draped fabric, patterns and belts.

Do you hate your bum?

Apparently there are four types of bottom shape. The results of a survey revealed that the ultimate bottom shape is an upside down heart shape, just like Jennifer Lopez's. Other celebrities who have this shape bottom are Kelly Brook and Dita Von Teese – the burlesque stripper.

The three other shapes revealed in the survey are V-shaped (wider up toward the hips), square and round.

Very few of us have that perfect bottom, but you should always check out your back view in the mirror to see how it looks in what you are wearing. Many of you may imagine you see a bigger bottom than you really have, but whatever size you imagine you see, you can help it to look better in the following ways:

> *I have days when I feel great and days when my arse won't fit into my jeans and I don't leave the house.*
> Kate Beckinsale

I have a large bottom with cellulite.

Keep away from clingy and smooth shiny fabrics.

Hold in, shapewear pants may give you more confidence.

I'd like to have a more curvaceous bum.

Apparently Penelope Cruz, in a movie, had to wear padding to create a larger bum as hers wasn't felt to be curvy enough, as did Jessica Simpson in the *Dukes of Hazard* TV series. Victoria Beckham's bum was digitally re-imaged to look bigger in the advertisements for the Beckhams' new perfume. You too could have a curvaceous derriere with 'contour pants'. It's cheaper than plastic surgery!

Do you like your legs?

I hate my 'tree trunk legs'.

Attract the eye to your best bits! Wear skirts that finish just below your knee at your slimmest part, or even a long skirt together with a top showing your fabulous décolleté. A wrap or tunic dress over soft drawstring or floppy trousers could be another way of concealing your legs. Always matte or opaque tights rather than patterned or shiny and never wear shoes with ankle straps as they give the illusion of shorter legs.

I have large thighs.

Clothes that drape and skim and never cling will flatter you, whilst looser, boot cut trousers work best to balance out your body shape.

I have short legs.

Trousers and jeans can be worn long over high heels and nude coloured shoes create the illusion of being an extension of your leg, so lengthening them.

I have long legs.

Lucky you!

I have skinny legs.

You can add the illusion of volume with textured, shiny, ribbed or coloured opaque tights.

Lighter-coloured or baggy trousers will also help your legs to look larger.

I have thin ankles.

You are one of the few that can wear ankle strap shoes and ankle boots.

I have fat ankles.

Never wear ankle straps, strappy shoes, ankle boots or crop trousers.

Do you have other dressing dilemmas?

I am pregnant.

You could either feel really sexy or just really large. If you have never had a bust before and suddenly you have cleavage, why not flaunt it now? Attract the eye to your new friends and detract from the baby bump. Showing skin, especially your décolleté, is sexy.

Wear off the shoulder tops to show flesh.

Wrap over style tops and dresses and soft, stretchy fabrics with elastane that hug your body work successfully if you are youthful and have remained toned and fit.

High-waisted, empire line dresses with a low-cut neckline will flatter and be sexy.

Underwear is also important and should be regularly checked for correct size and fit as your pregnancy progresses.

I have just had my baby and I don't look like those celebrity 'Yummy Mummies'.

Very few women are able to spring back into shape like the celebrities you see on all the pages of the magazines only two weeks after giving birth, with a flat tummy and wearing skimpy, British size eight clothes again. Most women take quite a few months and others years! So be realistic with your post-pregnancy wardrobe. Select an outfit you aim to wear in a month's time. You can always cheat a bit with body shaping underwear like the celebrities do on the red carpet. Gwyneth Paltrow admitted she wore Spanx hold in pants under her red carpet dresses after her pregnancies.

How can you look best on the beach?

You will need to get your body beach ready. Wax or laser unwanted hair on your legs, underarm and bikini line. Then exfoliate and moisturise ready for your fake tanning session.

Make sure your feet look great, with painted toenails and no hard skin (see Beauty section).

Once you have prepared your body and found that perfect swimsuit or bikini, you need to wear it with confidence, whilst being aware of your posture. You must stand up straight and hold your tummy and bottom in and pull up. Don't stoop to hide your big boobs or tummy. It will only make them look worse.

Wear a sarong or a sheer kaftan over your bikini or swimsuit when you need to walk anywhere. Better to look sexy and confident and discreetly covered up than to feel awkward.

Do you know which shape of bikini or swimsuit you look best in?

I have a boyish straight up and down shape.
You, like Cameron Diaz, are the shape that can wear any style bikini. Try small triangle cups or bandeau tops. If you have no bust you could always try a padded triangle top to add that little bit extra volume in the boob department. Bottoms can be 'boy short' style, high cut or tie side.

I have a pear shape.
If you are pear shaped like Jennifer Lopez, Kiera Knightly and Gwyneth Paltrow you can wear high legged bikinis that tie at the side, to create a less hippy, longer leg look. Padded tops, detailing, ruching and patterns are good illusion vehicles to create a bigger bust to balance out hips. Triangular halter

necks also work well. Just because you feel you have bigger hips or bum doesn't mean that the bikini should be bigger. Sometimes a smaller shaped bikini is more flattering.

I am curvy.
Kelly Brook and even Helen Mirren are the typical curvaceous body shapes that look best in a bikini that has wider straps for extra support, whilst also balancing out the body shape. Wiring and extra support within the framework of the bra top is important, so 50s style bikini shapes can work well for you. High cut bikini bottoms are the most flattering. Tankinis are also a good option for covering the tum. If you are wearing a swimsuit make sure the back is as low as possible. The higher the back and straighter cut the legs, the less flattering. There is also the 'miraclesuit', a swimsuit with corset control.

I have a large bust.
Even if your boobs aren't Dolly Parton-sized, the better the support in your bikini, the better your figure will look, as big boobs supported in the right place will create a longer torso and show off your waist. Take as much care with the fit of your bikini as you do your bra. After all more people are going to see you in it!

Jeans for your body shape

> *I wish I had invented blue jeans. They have expression, modesty, sex appeal, simplicity, all I can hope for in my clothes.*
>
> Yves Saint Laurent

Jeans are one of the most basic, yet essential items in our wardrobe and should work for our body shape whatever size we are. Naturally, nobody can help changing shape, putting on weight or ageing, but by dressing cleverly in the perfect pair of jeans, we can create the illusion of dropping a jeans size even if we actually haven't.

How can the correct fitting jeans really make a difference?

Light will always attract the eye, so make sure all faded or bleached areas are those which you wish the eyes to be attracted to. Fading is always better down the central sections of the jean leg (unless you are slim and wish to look curvier). Pockets and trims will attract the eye so strategic placing of pockets and their design is essential. If you have a small, flat bottom, choose a design that has large pockets with detailing. Higher placed pockets will give an instant bottom lift.

I have short legs.

If you are short-legged then wear heels with your jeans. If the boots or shoes are in view then keep them a neutral colour which will help blend into the background.

Prominent vertical stitching down side seams will lengthen legs Try to avoid too short jeans, cut-offs or turn ups – these create the illusion of shorter legs.

I'm an apple shape.

Apple shapes, or anyone who carries weight around their midriff and stomach, should look for slimmer cut jeans which show off their legs. If you have great legs you can carry off a narrower leg style. You can hide your midriff with a cleverly cut top, or something looser. Keep to a loose top and slim jeans, otherwise you will look like a shapeless sack! You are one of the few body shapes that can get away with wearing a paler wash or bleached jean together with a darker top to balance out your body shape. This will help to detract the eye from the midriff.

I'm a curvaceous body shape.

Dark coloured, boot cut shapes will be most flattering on larger thighs and pear shapes whilst slightly flared, boot cut legs will help balance curves. Lycra or elastane in denim will help gaping-waist-fit problems.

I'm a straight up and down body shape.

If you have a straight up and down figure with narrow hips,

then you can wear most jean shapes, however jeans with structure in a heavier denim will work best for you.

To add curves, choose jeans with styling details, pockets and bleached areas in strategic places which will attract the eye and create the illusion of a curvier body shape. If you have a longer body, wear a chunky wide belt on your hips.

I have heavy thighs.

Lycra content in denim has a little more stretch, giving you the chance to find a pair of jeans which fits both your hips as well as your thighs. If you're looking for a jean with roomy thighs and calves, wear styles which don't hug the body, such as a relaxed fit or boy cut or 'boyfriend' jean. Heavier weight denim will help conceal any lumps or bumps.

I have a short body.

If you have a short body and long legs, keep to wearing tonal colours with your jeans so as not to break up the body line. Wear your jeans very low slung as it will make your body appear longer.

I have a large bust.

If you have an ample bust and slim legs you can wear a light coloured jean and dark top to attract the eye away from being top heavy. Wear a fitted top and your jeans slim fitting to create maximum impact.

I am pear shaped.

Wear a dark jean and a light top to balance out your proportions. Make sure the pockets do not draw attention to the hips and wear thinner belts.

And remember...

Don't forget to look at your back view in the mirror – it's what others will see even if you can't. Designer jeans are usually cut very small and will vary from label to label, so don't be despondent about going up a size. You are more likely to feel bloated the week before your period, so for a 'feel good because you fitted into a size X or Y moment', don't shop for jeans that week.

   To keep your jeans looking their best, wash inside out in cold water to keep the dye colourfast.

I don't believe in the words fashion faux pas.

Christina Aguilera

I say, if you feel good with what you're doing,
let your freak flag fly.

Sarah Jessica Parker

I love Cate Blanchet because she gives everything she
wears a personal touch.

Valentino

Accessories – bags, hats and shoes

The correct accessories will "finish" an outfit. You can use accessories to compliment and tone in with your clothes – Nicole Kidman and Renee Zellweger use their accessories in this way – or as style statements using the latest colours and catwalk trends.

> *I used to have this horrible style. I had pink and white hair and had this giant papier-maché sea horse that rattled when I'd wear it on my back. Long skirts, eight scarves and bit of plastic...*
>
> Sienna Miller

Cleverly chosen accessories can completely change the look of old wardrobe favourites. Glamorous accessories can jazz up a little black dress. Stylish, beautiful leather bags and shoes can make a simple, inexpensive high street dress become part of a chic and expensive looking outfit. Flattering colourful scarves and jewellery worn near the face can reflect light to your skin and instantly give you a more youthful appearance.. The wrong accessories can also spoil an outfit by making it look cheap, busy or too contrived.

Q Is the bag you carry correct for your body shape and size?

I am a larger sized woman.

Larger women suit proportionally larger sized accessories.

I am a petite sized woman.

Smaller woman suit proportionally smaller handbags.

> " *I think better if I have a good hat on...* "
>
> Anna Piaggi

Q What style hat should you wear for your body shape?

A rule of thumb would be large woman, bigger hat, petite woman, smaller hat.

How can you balance out your face shape?

A hat should compliment your face shape. If you have a longish face, then the hat should have a good deep crown, balancing your face shape, otherwise it will give the appearance of being too flat on the head and make your face appear longer. Asymmetrical hats are very flattering to all face shapes. Upward tilting brims help lift and flatter the face to give a more youthful look, especially for the more mature woman.

Do your shoes suit you, however much you love them?

The shoes you wear are very important and can make or break an outfit.

Comfort is paramount and if you have sore feet then you will not be able to relax and enjoy yourself. Standing and walking well can give the illusion of instantly dropping pounds.

What height heel should I wear?

If you want to create the impression of longer legs, then go for a higher heel worn with trousers. If your feet hurt wearing high heels, try placing gel pads under the ball of the foot.

Don't wear very high heels with very short skirts and low cut tops.

Flat shoes such as ballet pumps are, of course, the most comfortable, but do not give the impression of longer legs. A kitten heel is more flattering than a completely flat shoe.

What shape shoe is best for my legs?

Try out shoe styles and evaluate the effect on your leg shape in the mirror- just as you would a dress. Do not buy a shoe just because you love its styling- it may just not suit you! Ankle straps and ankle boots are only flattering for very long legs with slim ankles. Few of us sadly have legs like that! Strappy sandals can be flattering as long as the straps are not too heavy.

If you are going to wear sandals, then your feet must be well cared for. There is nothing worse than nice shoes on badly tended feet.

What boot is best for my legs?

Make sure that you don't have any flesh hanging over the top of your knee high boots. The most flattering length boot is one that ends just above the widest part of your calf.

Only wear an ankle boot with a skirt if you have very slim, perfect legs like Kate Middleton. If you do wear them, team them with opaque tights so they become less obvious. A shoe boot that sits lower under the ankle is more flattering than an ankle boot. High flat boots such as a riding boot style look great with most outfits..

I have wide feet.

If you have wide feet and bigger legs, try a less delicate shoe, not one necessarily with a round toe, but one that has a slightly thicker heel, even a wedge. The lower cut the front of the shoe, the more flattering it will be for your legs. There are shoes that are made in wider styles. You can find them in specialist shops online.

I have big feet.

Don't despair. The average model foot size is never less than a British size 7½ or 8, European size 41/42. If your feet are bigger than this then you can find styles to fit you on the Internet and also at a few specialised shops. If you are very conscious of your big feet, don't buy shoes that make a statement. Choose a neutral colour like beige to be less noticeable.

Can I match my shoes with my outfit?

It's always better if you are making a bold statement with colour to not go the whole hog. Less is always more. A red dress is great, but not necessarily worn with red shoes too. It is important to have a selection of shoe styles that coordinate with your various outfits as the perfect shoe will make an outfit and the wrong shoe make everything look wrong-old fashioned, too business like or too evening.

> *If diamonds are not a girl's best friend,*
> *then it must be boys.*
>
> Paloma Picasso

Q Do you know how to accessorise with jewellery?

I would love to wear proper jewellery but can't afford it.
You don't have to be able to afford diamonds to add some 'bling' to your outfits.

It is very easy nowadays to buy a key piece of jewellery that really creates the finishing touch. This jewellery can be cheap and cheerful and from the high street, flea market or car boot sale. It's all about how you wear it. The trick about wearing cheap jewellery is to not pretend that it's real, but to wear it with panache. Wear more than one bangle to make a statement. If it's pearls make them big and multi-stranded.

Are there jewellery rules?
A simple rule of accessorising would be busy dress, plain jewellery, plain dress, busy jewellery.

So what would you wear with a little black dress (LBD)?
You will need to decide if you are going for ladylike, demure and classic; or funky with some brightly coloured or interesting quirky jewels. Your choice of how you wear your jewellery can completely change the look of the dress.

For example, classic elegant jewellery will say exactly that about you, but if you take any classic item and wear it in an edgy or unexpected way you will appear younger and more stylish. If you wear a small diamante brooch discretely, as though it were an expensive diamond heirloom, it will just look as though you tried, but couldn't afford the real thing. But if you wear the same piece together with a second brooch making more of a statement, it will say you meant it to be fun and fake.

Be brave and break the rules with accessories – it's one of the few times that you can.

Your wardrobe

So, let's have a look through your wardrobe.
Do you wear all your clothes?

I look in my wardrobe everyday and, although I have lots of clothes, find that I have nothing to wear.
Your clothing has to suit your lifestyle and everything you own should work hard to earn its place in your wardrobe.

It's not necessary to replace or update your wardrobe each season unless you are super-rich or a fashion victim, but it is necessary to check through your wardrobe for clothes that are:

- Too big for you.
- Too small for you.
- Unfashionable by 20 years, but definitely not 'vintage'.
- Tired and worn.
- Stained.
- Unfashionable/past their sell-by date

All of the above should be repaired, cleaned or relegated to charity or second hand shops to leave space for the clothes that actually fit you, suit your *current* size and body shape and life you lead. It is no point having a wardrobe full of suits if you no longer work in an office. If you live in the countryside now, town clothes are unlikely to be worn on a daily basis and if you are with your kids most of the day, then you require child-friendly clothes for the daytime and something to dress up in to feel a bit sexy and glamorous in for your husband or partner on your important "date" evenings out with him.

> *People who find fashion strange or trivialising are missing the point. Pride in yourself and the way you look does not convey or cover up any deficiency.*
>
> Baroness Susan Greenfield, scientist

So why do you never wear some of your clothes?

They don't suit me.

By now, you should have looked in the mirror to understand your body shape and colouring. You may still see yourself as a different size from your true size and still have self-esteem issues, but you should be able to understand more clearly how to dress for your *best* you.

Try on everything in your wardrobe and imagine that I am there with you, helping you be really analytical, even critical, but *not* harsh on yourself. Ask yourself what you feel about this outfit and how you *really* look in it. Ask yourself what is it doing for you. How is the colour for your colouring? How is the neckline? Look at your back view. How is it? Look at the length where the skirt hem finishes on your legs and the sleeve length. Are they both good for you? Do the trousers skim over your body? Does the cut flatter?

Be really truthful to yourself.

Step outside yourself and try to see yourself as others would see you. Look at yourself from all angles. It is important not to forget your back view and profile. You are a three dimensional person and you are seen from all sides. Not just the front. *Do not* just focus on the most disliked part of you, such as your tummy. See the whole of you and the positive. Ask yourself truthfully, is it making you look your best?

If the answer is no, then it has to go. You only want a wardrobe full of clothes you actually wear, that work and mix and match together, that suit you and that you really love. It would be better to have a few that you really do wear than masses of clothes that you never wear.

Don't throw these unwanted clothes away, but create piles of them to give to charity, or to sell at your local nearly new clothes shop, on eBay, or at your local car boot sale.

It was a bargain so I bought it.
When you go sales shopping, go with a specific shopping list

in mind of what you need to buy to add to your current wardrobe. Either aim to buy wardrobe basics such as a classic coat, trousers, little black dress etc, or make a list of the gaps in your wardrobe. Do you need a perfect pair of black trousers? Do you not have a top that goes with your favourite skirt? Do you have a dress that you never wear because you don't have any shoes that go with it? Do you have a wardrobe full of clothes but nothing that works together?

Only buy what you really need. Do not buy that must-have bargain, even if it was £2,000 reduced to £20! A bargain isn't a bargain if it doesn't suit you, fit you or work in your wardrobe. And don't buy it with the thought that you'll wear it when you lose weight. Live in the moment and buy it to wear now. When you shop, wear appropriate underwear that will work under the intended outfit (for example a plunge evening bra if you are shopping for an evening dress) and take a pair of heels to try things on with.

I thought I liked it but I don't think it suits me.
Now that you are aware of what works for you, your body shape and colouring, you can be more discerning about your past wardrobe choices. Did you buy a dress because you thought it was a pretty style? But does the colour really work for your skin tones? Did you buy a sweater only because the colour went with your favourite trousers? Does the sweater have a polo neck that makes you look larger, now that you know that you look better in a V-neck? Have you looked at your back view in that pencil skirt? Are you seeing cellulite as

the fabric is too sheer? Is that shirt straining at the buttons over your bosom? Is the neckline of the T-shirt you wear all the time the wrong shape for you? Do you keep buying baby pink items when actually you look better in a shade of coral pink? Imagine I am there asking you all these sorts of questions and be ruthless with your clothes. Remember this is the beginning of the new you.

> *A woman's dress should be like a barbed wire fence.*
> *Serving its purpose without obstructing the view.*
> Sophia Loren

I bought it out of desperation.

Do you wait to shop for that outfit you need for that special occasion at the last minute? Is this because you are waiting to lose weight and hate how you look at the moment? Do you feel embarrassed about how you look in the mirror and feel that you will be judged by the shop assistants? Do you think you won't find anything suitable in your size? Do you not know how and where to start? Do you hate shopping? If lack of money is your problem you can shop at places like Primark or any of the Supermarkets where you can pick up the latest looks for only a few pounds.

If you are shopping for a last minute outfit, be focused and have in mind the look you would like to achieve, even if you are not happy with your current body shape. It's about making the best of yourself now – not in the future. Is there something in your wardrobe already existing that you can update with new accessories – new shoes, bag, belt or jewellery? Does it need altering, adding new buttons, new zip, shortening, lengthening, taking in, letting out, repairing or dry-cleaning?

It was a spur of the moment purchase.
Most boutiques and stores will take your purchases back within 28 days and give you a refund as long as you have your receipt and the clothes are pristine and unworn. So if you get it home and realise that it really doesn't make you look your best, for any reason – take it back. You don't have to explain – just say it is unsuitable. The retailers are not going to love me for reminding you of your rights, but much better that you don't waste your money on clothes that are only going to hang unworn in your wardrobe.

It's too big for me now.
So you have lost weight and your clothes are now too big for you. Some can be altered at your local dry cleaners and others will be too complicated to start playing around with as it may cost more to alter and re-make than to buy again new. Once you start altering some styles, the proportions become out of sync.

Check the fit. Do the shoulders hang off your shoulders? It is essential that these fit correctly. Do you need to bring in the shoulder seams? Can you take in with darts or extra seams? If you take in the waist band of a skirt or trousers what is the impact of the alteration on the fit around your bottom? Consider all these things before you commission the alteration, as however good it is, it may completely change the look and the original styling of the item.

It's too small for me now.

If you really are certain that you are going to fit into this item of clothing again one day, not in the too distant future, then I will allow you to put it on the top shelf for the celebratory day you reach your target weight... but... does it actually suit you if and when it fits again?

Is the colour good for you? Is it something that works with the rest of your wardrobe? Do you *need* it? There is a difference between *want* and *need*.

> *If I feel good in something – like I could run a marathon in it – I'll wear it.*
>
> Kate Hudson

I don't feel comfortable in it.

Comfortable doesn't only mean how something fits – too loose or too tight – but how you feel in it. Do you feel uncomfortable because the neck is low and you think you may be exposing too much cleavage? Do you worry about your back view? Do you hate your knees or calves and the dress finishes just in the wrong place? Maybe subconsciously you know the colour or pattern doesn't suit you so you feel uncomfortable. To look and feel great in your clothes you must feel comfortable, inside and out. You should feel confident and sexy in your outfit – because you know it works for your colouring and body shape.

I thought I'd keep it for sentimental reasons.

Are you too old to wear it now? Could the outfit be a mutton dressed as lamb syndrome? Is it old fashioned rather than something that you could bring out again to wear as 'vintage'. It is always nice to keep clothes for sentimental reasons, whether it is to pass down to your children, grandchildren or just to have for a memory, but if you are keeping it to wear again, then look at it and then at yourself and see if the two still match.

My partner or husband bought it for me.

If your partner or husband really cares and understands you, he should welcome the fact that you are re-evaluating the inner and outer you, as the likelihood is that not only you will benefit but so will he *and* your relationship together. So if you feel bad that he bought it for you and now you are getting rid of it, then explain why it doesn't suit you *any longer* so that he will understand and buy you something next time that suits you and that you feel sexy and wonderful in when you are out together.

> *I try to mix ladylike sweetness*
> *with really sexy vampiness.*
>
> Jennifer Lopez

It's too sexy for me.

Do you want to wear clothes that make you invisible and that do not draw any attention to you?

Do you feel that if you wear a low neckline showing some cleavage, it becomes too sexy?

If you are wearing a dress that reveals cleavage, it is best not to show leg above the knee, especially if you are of a certain age, however good your legs are.

But if you have a good bust, why not show a little of it off? It will attract the eye and detract from all the other bits of you that you dislike.

If you grew up having a larger bust than your school friends and became conscious at an early age how eye contact in conversation hovers there rather than on your face, you may wish to cover up more as it's now a habit to do so. But a hint of cleavage won't automatically attract men's eyes. You body shape will look better, too, with some flesh on show.

> *The body is meant to be seen, not all covered up.*
> Marilyn Monroe

> *I wouldn't feel right wearing clothes that*
> *covered my whole body.*
> Christina Aguilera

I don't feel sexy in it.
Sometimes classic styles can make you look old before your time. Avoid blouses with bows, boxy suits, tweeds and anything that's too severe. A classic style can be made to look sexier if worn in an unexpected way. Maybe accessorised with a contrasting colour. Maybe with a flash of lingerie lace.

Maybe a denim jacket or a leather biker jacket over a silk dress. A pair of sexy shoes. Lovely lingerie worn simply for your own pleasure will also make you feel sexy. It doesn't matter if no-one else will see it. It's how you feel about yourself.

I keep putting it on but never wear it as I don't seem to feel right in it.

Is it the colour that is too pale, too dark or the wrong tone against your skin? Or is it the cut that doesn't work well for your body shape. If you have an item of clothing that has hung in your wardrobe unworn, get rid of it. Replace it with something that works.

You should not have to try on lots of outfits that are discarded across the bedroom before venturing out of the house!

> *I leave notes saying I apologize for the state of the closet. I'll clean it up.*
> Sarah Jessica Parker

I don't have anything to go with it.

Try it on and decide what style, shape and colour you need to buy to coordinate with this item. When you go shopping take it with you so that you can colour match it and also see if everything works together. Sometimes something that looks good in the shop doesn't really work how you thought it would when you get home. It might be also that the sales assistant was very enthusiastic and persuasive.

Wardrobe tips

You should treat your clothes with care and they will last better. It doesn't matter whether they are cheap or expensive; give them the same attention.

You should:

- Always air your clothes after wearing.
- Check your clothes for stains and ideally wash or dry clean after wearing before putting them back in the wardrobe.
- Iron them after washing, before putting them away in your wardrobe. That way you'll always have something to wear in the morning.
- Check for fallen hems, missing buttons.
- Don't wear the same pair of shoes every day. Rotate them so that they get aired and don't smell.
- Clean your shoes and mend worn down heels.
- Keep your clothes hanging on non-wire hangers so they keep their shape.

Shopping tips

- Make your wardrobe shopping a battle plan, not a whim.
- Make a list of what you really need not want.
- Make a list of what you have in your wardrobe that have no coordinating items
- Make a list of what items need accessories: belts, shoes, jewellery, cardigans.
- Do you already have the wardrobe basics or do you need to buy them? Great black trousers, LBD, white shirt, a jacket, skirt, day dress, evening dress, evening cover up etc.

- Only buy what you can fit into now. Not if or when, but today.

- Only buy a jacket if it does up. Don't say 'I'll wear it open'.

- Don't buy a top only to wear under something. Each item needs to be able to stand alone.

- Don't shop when you've been for a long, boozy lunch.

- Check that you can return the item if you are not confident about your purchase.

- Wear comfortable shoes to shop in and take a pair of heels to try on with.

- Wear underwear that supports well and works under evening wear as well as day wear.

- If a dress or a jacket needs more than three areas of alteration, don't buy it.

Dressing appropriately for an occasion

The job interview
I don't know what to wear.

You have 30 seconds to create that crucial first impression. Find out exactly what employees are likely to wear in the workplace of the job you are going up for. If it is a casual, younger style workplace, you could find the approach to dressing is more casual, with jeans and T-shirts being the norm, or no dress code at all. In a company where the men wear suits and ties, you will need to dress in a similar vein as there is likely to be a dress code. Dress as though you are already working in the company. When you work for a company, and you are client facing, you are the "face" of that brand.

I haven't got anything suitable.
You don't have to wear a suit to look professional. It is all about looking appropriate. Clean, tidy and groomed is the most important. Clothes that look tired, dirty and unkempt with buttons hanging off or hems falling down and faded areas are not appropriate. Make sure your shoes are clean and polished and that your heels are not worn down. Trainers are generally not suitable but neither are spiky stilettos.

I am too fat to get in my old work clothes now.
I would suggest looking for a flattering outfit that fits you well now, with a soft shape. Try layering, leaving a longer length shirt loose under an unstructured jacket or cardigan. A pair of medium height heels, not flats. A good handbag is important. Although structured tailoring flatters most figure shapes, office work wear has now evolved to softer tailoring and separates.

The new job
How can I dress to look my best in my work?
How *you* look influences your client's view of the company. Dress appropriately, especially if you have client facing meetings. Good grooming is also important. You should have a stylish haircut, or at least clean and tidy hair. Wear some make-up so that you look as though you take care of your appearance and make sure that your nails are clean, and not

too long. A recent survey acknowledged that women who wear makeup in the workplace are more likely to be promoted

I would still like my personality to show.
Corporate dressing doesn't have to be boring. Interesting accessories add the finishing touches to all outfits. Even a watch can say volumes about you (see accessories section).

Can I wear skirts or dresses?
Try mixing and matching jackets and skirts. A jacket and skirt can look as smart as a suit, while a dress can look business-like and elegant too. A dress with a crisp fabric and tailoring, such as a belted shirt-dress, would be better than a wrap dress. Plain rather than printed is probably more appropriate for office wear. Cotton, cashmere or lambswool cardigans will look more suitable than chunky country knits.

I don't want to look too sexy.
I have frequently come across female employees who have wished to be only seen for the work they do, not be seen as a woman in the workplace by their male colleagues. The women's solution was to wear 'shapeless' sexless clothing. But you can still look feminine in the workplace without looking overtly sexy. Wear clothes that skim the body, not cling, and that flatter your shape without being revealing. It's all about being appropriate – a skirt that's not too short, a blouse that's not too tight across the bust or undone too low and outfits that look professional.

I work from home.

Try to get dressed each day, out of your tracky bottoms or pyjamas, even if it's only into jeans and a T-shirt. It will make you feel more motivated.

Casual

What does 'casual' on a party invitation mean?

Dress to look good in chic but comfortable dressed-down style, not full-on party mode. Maybe jeans, high heels and a sexy or smart top. It's not about stilettos and sexy evening dresses, but mixing relaxed style with a touch of glamour.

If I am asked to wear 'smart business casual', what does it mean?

Smart business casual is generally a relaxed jacket and trousers or cardigan, shirt and skirt; a combination equivalent to a men's suit worn without a tie. The impression you give off must say you are above all professional, authoritative, you know what you are doing, you are efficient, and also well-groomed.

What does 'smart casual' on a party invite mean?

Simple but elegant. Not jeans, shorts, or anything you'd wear on a day to day basis or for work. You need to look as though you've made an effort. For daytime, it could be a dress, a beautifully cut pair of trousers and a top. Linen works well for summer, although it creases, or crisp white cotton, which you could mix and match with some colour. For evening, again you could wear a dress, that Little Black Dress or the wrap dress that works for all body shapes. Anything in silk is always a good classic wardrobe staple. Any fabric that is sensual to the touch will look more elegant. Shoes should be elegant and a high heel makes an outfit more evening.

The dinner party invite

I don't want to be underdressed – but equally don't want to be overdressed.

Do you know what any of the other guests are wearing? Ask the hostess or a friend who is going what she is wearing.

Mix understated with glam such as silk or lace top with jeans.

Dress down a cocktail style dress with low-key styling such as a suede, leather or denim jean style jacket.

Or accessorise up a simple little dress (you can always sneak off to the loo to remove the accessories).

The cocktail party

The invite didn't have a dress code suggested – I have no idea what to wear.

If you wear something classic you can never go wrong, or look out of place. Don't go down the jeans and evening top route. You don't know how dressed up the other women there may be. The little black dress is always the safe option. Cocktail party style is sexy but elegant, feminine and ladylike.

> *Too much of a good thing can be wonderful.*
> Mae West

The black tie event

Black tie no longer means that a long dress is a must. A knee length or longer cocktail dress can be appropriate too. It is also very chic to wear a beautifully cut female version of the tuxedo suit teamed with very high sexy heels, and a lace or silk camisole underneath.

Men, though, will always find a dress sexier. Be comfortable in what you wear. You will have a miserable evening if your shoes are too high and your dress too tight. Remember you will also need to sit down and eat at some point in the evening. It's always worth doing a phone around to other women you know who are invited. You can then check what they are wearing If you want to stand out, wear a colour, as so many wear black,

> *I hate stealing the show, but I'd worn a lot of black, covering up things, and I thought – not this year.*
>
> Kate Winslet
>
> when she wore the red Ben de Lisi dress at the Oscars

I can't afford a new dress.

'Black tie' doesn't have to mean a new dress but it does mean *dress up*. Dressing up in my opinion means looking glamorous, elegant and sexy and "finished" (with painted nails, hair washed and blow-dried, with a bit of extra grooming effort). Even if you have worn the same dress before, you could change the look of it with different jewellery, accessories and shoes. No one will ever notice, especially if you look wonderful in it. They'll only notice you looking your best. If you feel good in a dress why not wear it again? Lots of celebrities recycle their clothes, especially old favourites. Even Princess Anne is known for the constant recycling of her wardrobe.

> *The only rule is don't be boring and dress cute wherever you go. Life is too short to blend in.*
>
> Paris Hilton

How can I find underwear to make the most of my figure under my clinging, revealing dress?

To look sexy in your long dress, remember how to dress for your body shape and make the most of your curves, attracting the eye to the bits you like and distracting from those you don't. If you have great legs, find a long dress with a slit on the leg. If you have good shoulders, go for a one shouldered Grecian style or strapless. And of course there is always a backless dress option. But don't forget to wear supportive lingerie under your chosen dress to give your body a great shape.

> *Any model or Hollywood actress who wears fancy designer ball gowns knows how to expertly manipulate gaffer tape to mush, lift and hold your breasts like a bra. It's a perfect temporary boob job. When you wear those complicated, low-cut dresses, and you're 40, that's how you can achieve perfect cleavage.*
>
> Teri Hatcher

I am worried about my outfit.

Before you leave home and you have decided on your outfit, check yourself in front of the mirror. Does the dress fit? Is your underwear hidden? Is your dress revealing too much when you lean forward or walk or just move? Do you need toupée-tape (double-sided tape) to stick the revealing parts of your dress to your body as the celebrities do for the red carpet? Or do you need control pants to hold those lumps and bumps in?

> *I like to move fast, and wearing high heels was tough, and low heels with a skirt is unattractive. So pants took over.*
>
> Katharine Hepburn

I am not very good at walking in heels as I usually wear flats.
Are your shoes new or have you road-tested them before? Can you actually last an evening in them without serious pain? Comfortable feet equal a great night. If they are very high, have you ever tried party feet gel inserts for under the balls of your feet? Better to be comfortable and be able to walk with confidence and ease than totter, especially after a few drinks.

I would like to look glamorous.
Glamour is about really *owning* your look. It's about feeling drop dead gorgeous, and feeling and looking sexy. You don't have to be wearing a revealing dress that lets it all hang out –
– but the dress always has to be worn with confidence, great

posture and attitude. Glamour gets noticed; you cannot be invisible if you are glamorous. Glamour catches the eye. It shows off your curves. It makes other women jealous.

Always dress for you. If you feel good then you will look good to others.

Part Three

Being Your Best You

· · · · · · · · · · · ·

How you feel about the new you and how you can continue on the journey

The third stage and final part of your journey

> *Right now you are one choice away from a new beginning – one that leads you toward becoming the fullest human being you can be.*
>
> Oprah Winfrey

By now you should have asked yourself questions and found the answers. You will have looked in the mirror and seen yourself as others see you and should be looking at a brand new reflection of yourself. One that is more confident and optimistic.

You've soul searched in Part One of your journey, and learnt tricks to improve the physical you in Part Two. Part Three is all about putting yourself out there in your 'new you' mind and body and see who appears.

You are now aware of how to make the best of your face and body shape with clothes, beauty products and quick fixes. You may not have implemented any changes yet, but you are ready to do so. The most important thing is being in the mindset to make those changes. You should no longer be putting off the diet and exercise if required until another day.

You approach everything now with a positive attitude. If you are happy in your own skin, and more accepting, you will exude energy and optimism. You don't have to change your face or your body, all you have to change is how you see yourself. You are now standing at the crossroads of your new life and need confidence to go out and get.

So how are you going to really change your life? What are you going to do about getting out again, creating new relationships and maybe a new social circle of friends? How are you going to start having a more vibrant social life? Maybe finding that new job and re-starting your working life? Discovering the new you.

> *Anyone's life truly lived consists of work, sunshine, exercise, soap, plenty of fresh air, and a happy contented spirit.*
>
> Lillie Langtry

> *Real enthusiasm comes from the heart and ignites the whole system. If you have that, there's no resistance, nothing to sabotage your actions. You can succeed at almost anything.*
>
> Anita Roddick

So how are you going to kick-start your new social life?

Is your life like being on the treadmill? Can you never find time to get out of your home or your office? If you want to really change your life, it's important to find a balance between your daytime 'job' and your 'you' time. Your daytime job encompasses everything from being a mum and doing the housework and chores to whatever paid daytime job you may have.

Your 'you' time could include getting out to exercise, even if it's only a short walk; taking up a hobby; getting out to a place where you can socialise and meet friends or make new friends. You need an activity that is for *you* only.

So where do you go for your 'you' time and how do you make new friends?

Work out your priorities and the people you *really* want to be with. Health should be your number one priority, family the second, and friends the third.

'You time' suggestions

- Try Voluntary work. Helping others always makes you feel good.
- Try www.csv.org.uk; www.timebank.org.uk.
- Go for a walk.
- Try learning a new sport.
- Try learning a new skill, language, art, singing, cooking.
- Delegate some more at work.
- Pamper yourself. Try essential oils in the bath or go for a massage.

What celebrities do for their 'Me time'

Kate Winslet

'I love a night at home in front of the telly. I'm in that dressing gown and love it. I'm all for comfort and being cosy.'

Shakira Caine

'I swim religiously. Every day if possible. When things get too much, when I feel I can't cope, I swim for an hour. It's important to find out what you can do to relieve stress, and how to cope with it.'

Sandra Bullock

'On my ranch in Texas I can recharge my batteries and revel

in doing absolutely nothing, just watch the grass grow, enjoy the sunset and see friends.'

Mary Nightingale
'Pruning and digging in my garden gives me the greatest feeling of relaxation and calm. I get a real sense of satisfaction when I see the results of my hard work. A sunny afternoon with the secateurs and a large spade – heaven!'

Demi Moore
'I like being physical and being out and about. I spend a lot of time going to the park, the zoo or the beach with the kids and taking bike rides.'

Joanna Lumley
'Deal with stress by breaking anxieties down into small manageable areas. Always give yourself rewards, like a nice cup of coffee, during a stressful day.'

Making new friends

I don't know where to start.
You need to get out of the house to meet new people. Whether you live in the town or the countryside, there will always be somewhere that is the heart and soul of your local community.

How do I begin?

If you live out of town, and you don't know anyone else in the area, you need to take up an activity where you will meet other men and women. Obviously in a big city there will be more choice as you only have to look in your local paper or in the window of the newsagent or library to find out what's happening locally to you. And of course there is the Internet to search on. If you live in the countryside, there may only be the local village post office, village shop or village hall, but that is where you will hear all the local gossip and what's happening where.

So where are you going to go? And what activity would you now like to learn?

> *I refuse to join any club that would have me as a member.*
> Groucho Marx

Some places to make new friends

- Health club
- Exercise class
- Tennis club
- Dancing classes
- Cooking class
- Art class
- Bridge club
- Coffee shops

- Art galleries
- Weight watchers
- Local evening classes of any sort
- Dog walks
- Local supermarket!

I'm shy.

Are you too shy to go out on your own and join a class? Do you think that others will be judging you or is it because you won't know anyone? But the others may not know anyone either. So have a go and imagine everyone else to be as shy as you. Look out for someone else who is standing on their own and be brave and strike up a conversation with them. They will be eternally grateful to you, as they may have had even less confidence than you. A brave face often covers huge insecurities.

Did you always want to learn to paint or play bridge? Now's your chance. There are a myriad classes in which you could enrol and meet other, like-minded women.

If you live in town, the world is your oyster for places to go and things to do and you will be spoilt for choice. But although there are so many choices, it doesn't mean that anyone is actually going to talk to you there. So you need to choose your activity carefully, an activity that involves interaction with your fellow classmates in pairs or groups. It could be as sedentary or energetic as you please. It's not really about the activity. It's more about meeting and mixing with new groups of people.

You could always have a regular skinny latte at your local coffee shop. Drink in – not take out. You may find that there are interesting daily regular visitors there too.

So you've now joined a club and are going out and about to new activities, but you find that you are still not really able to relate to people properly.

Is it your body language that is putting them off? Why do some people manage to attract others to them like moths to a light and others stand on their own, even if they are good looking?

> *Think sexy and confident. It all starts in the head.*
>
> Ivana Trump

What is charisma?
The word charisma is from the ancient Greek word *kharis*, meaning gift, as if you were seen to be charismatic, the Gods would have breathed a special gift of the spirit into you. So how do you become charismatic? It's about having a magnetism and aura that compels you to be noticed. There is no reason why you can't develop from being an introverted person to an extroverted one.

There is a difference between just 'being present' in a room and feeding off others' energy, and creating your own energy source which will draw others in to you. It's about being an upbeat and confident person, with body language to match. It's about the attitude you present to the world.

Men and women who have charisma use eye contact to engage with you. This indicates that you are the 'chosen one' and that they find you fascinating. This makes you feel good as all focus is on you. A person you find yourself attracted to will leave you in a 'feel good' state as they gave you their undivided attention. Successful charmers have positivity and are skilled at expressing and transmitting these positive emotions to others.

But don't you have to be really pretty?
A charismatic person isn't necessarily the best looking but one who generates a magnetic energy. The power of attraction is about fooling others into thinking that you are the most interesting, gorgeous person in the room. This is not about twiddling hair strands or getting out that cleavage but drawing people into your aura. Be intriguing and charismatic and attentive to your admirers. Make them think that you are the best listener in the world and nothing matters at that moment other than what they are telling you. Even if it is absolute rubbish!

> *We all lose our looks eventually. Better develop your character and interest in life... Character contributes to beauty. It fortifies a woman as her youth fades. A mode of conduct, a standard of courage, discipline, fortitude, and integrity can do a great deal to make a woman beautiful.*
> Jacqueline Bisset

How can I become charismatic?

- Accept yourself and your faults. This makes others feel comfortable with you as they can identify with your faults too. No one's perfect.
- Try to relax and be at ease, it will make others feel at ease too. Try to hide your tensions and stress.
- Be open to meeting new people and always with a positive attitude. Be interested in them, even if you are not. You may be pleasantly surprised.
- Smile. It changes others' attitude to you.
- Be optimistic, a glass half-full person. You will find that this is infectious. Others are drawn to the confident, optimistic person, not the shy and frightened individual, slouching in the corner.
- Be calm. Don't forget to breathe and if you find yourself breathing very fast, try to take some deep breaths to slow your breathing down.

Your body language tells all about you to others.

You can use it to show others how you feel and to read how others react to you. So if you are shy, lacking in confidence and have low-self esteem, override your mental thoughts and think about the physical you that is being shown to the world.

> *When I was 25 I was so lacking in self-esteem that I didn't have the confidence to enjoy my fame or shine socially. I never felt able to really let myself go, because I was so worried what the man would think.*
>
> Fiona Fullerton

How can I make a good first impression?

- Don't smile nervously and automatically at everyone you meet. Be slower with your smiles and make the person you are meeting aware that your smile is fully intended just for them. Make them feel special.

- Encourage the people you are meeting to talk about themselves. Pay attention and wait for them to finish their answers.

- The best way for getting people to talk is 'reciprocal disclosure'. Reveal something about yourself and the other person is likely to respond with a similar disclosure.

- Concentrate and don't look distracted and over their shoulder.

- Try to match and emulate the pace and volume of speech of your companion.

- Don't be hostile or argumentative.

- Be aware of how people react to you. Do you still have a connection or are they avoiding eye contact or looking bored? If so, why? Are you talking too fast, or is it all about you?

- Don't invade the other person's personal space. You can mirror their movements, so if they lean in, so can you.

- Everyone has something to offer. Especially you. So don't try too hard to be liked, but try harder to be more open to liking others and you will find others warming more to you.

I feel self-conscious when I walk into a party.
How are you walking into a room? Do you walk with a confidence and assuredness, holding yourself tall? Conjure up an imaginary friend at the end of the room, preferably near the bar and walk purposefully towards this area where you can stop and collect yourself again. Even if you didn't need a drink, it gave you a reason to walk in that direction too. Once you have your drink you can scan the room to see who you might know or who you'd like to get to know. Your outer shell of confidence will bring others to talk to you, whilst you stand there. Always look happy and upbeat. A miserable looking person will be ignored.

I feel self-conscious when I am meeting someone new.
Are you standing with your arms crossed or leaving them loose at your sides? Crossing your arms creates a protection around you, a barrier. You should appear to look open and friendly. Not closed and wary. When you are meeting someone for the first time, do you sit in a relaxed and attentive way or in a frightened and defensive way? You may not even realise that you are doing this. You will often find that you are mirroring the person whom you are relating to. You may find that you are both sitting in the same way and

doing the same things with your arms. You will certainly find this happening if you are flirting. But it can happen everywhere, even at a job interview.

I need to appear confident at my job interview.
Eye contact and openness is very important when being interviewed. As an interviewee, you will not get on well if you are perceived to be hiding something by never looking your prospective boss in the face. You may also find that if you mirror your interviewer's body language you could seem too relaxed. Remember to sit with your legs crossed if wearing a skirt.

It doesn't matter how good you may be at your job or look in your interview clothes if you don't have the correct body language at the interview. Don't invade the interviewer's personal space. Don't be manic with your gesticulations or enthusiasm, and don't cross your arms as this can be perceived as defensive. Sit up and be poised and collected.

The first date

What impression do you want to give?

I want to appear sexy but not too sexy. How should I dress?
Your date wants to go on a night out with *you,* not your outfit. Make sure that your outfit is appropriate for the person you are meeting with and the location.

- Don't go for too sexy, too skimpy, too short, too much cleavage, too tight. In fact 'too' anything is out. (Men want to look at other women wearing not too much – not the one that they are with, in case everyone else is looking at her for that reason too.)
- A man wants to be proud of the date that he is out with – not embarrassed.
- If you are wearing something with some cleavage revealed cover up the rest.
- You could always reveal your shoulders or back. They can be just as sexy.
- Don't wear anything that you need to constantly adjust or fiddle with.
- You want to look uncontrived, as though you threw the outfit together (stylishly), even if you really took three days agonising over what to wear.
- A skirt or a dress will make you feel more feminine.
- If you're really not a dress person, then go for a sexy evening style top teamed with jeans.
- And if you want to feel sexy without dressing to be obvious, then just wear some sexy undies under your simple, understated outfit. He will never know – well maybe not on that first date anyway!

I would like to look like the woman he'd want to marry.
This is not just about what you are wearing but how you conduct yourself. If you really want to be with this man, then you have to be *you*. So is the 'you' that you are showing this

man the real one? Or is it an act? No one can sustain the act of being someone they aren't for any length of time. And if you do, you are not being true to yourself or to your prospective partner. A good relationship is based on truth.

I don't know how to look self-confident.
It's all about body language. How you hold yourself. How you walk, hold your head up, use your hands and gestures and how you stand. Think about being tall and proud. Try to have your facial expressions, arms and hands as relaxed as possible.

I have forgotten how to flirt for fun.
Have you forgotten how to flirt, or do you flirt with everyone, even your own sex? Flirting is fun and can attract admirers to you. Flirting is all about body language and eye contact.
Do you make eye contact, or do you studiously avoid catching anyone's eye? Eyes tell you everything about how you, or someone else feels: happy, sad, lonely, excited, sexy or scared. This is also why if you fancy someone you look into their eyes. This is why you tend to not engage eye contact with strangers, in case it makes them want to start up an unwanted dialogue, or you give off the wrong signals. But if you do want to start up a dialogue or a flirt, you do so, by engaging eye contact, even across a room. Some people are scared of eye contact but others may feel that if you are prepared to look them back in the eye you are honest and up front and confident.

How can I seduce him into thinking I'm wonderful?

To charm is to seduce and you can seduce not only for sex, but to 'lure' others into your 'friendship fold'. If you have created a scenario where you have charmed someone into feeling at ease with you, then you may also have created a feeling of intimacy and warmth. Flattery, eye contact, light flirtation and making someone feel good about themselves are the keys..

Q Can you work on and improve your existing relationship?

Maybe you already have a partner with whom you are dissatisfied, and the relationship is less than perfect.

> *Ideally, couples need three lives; one for him, one for her, and one for them together.*
>
> Jacqueline Bisset

> *I want a man who's kind and understanding. Is that too much to ask of a millionaire?*
>
> Zsa Zsa Gabor

I grew up with the idea that my perfect man would be out there somewhere.

Are your expectations in love too high? Did you grow up with the notion that you would meet your knight in shining armour who would whisk you away on his white charger into the sunset and then you would both live happily ever after?

> *If you want to sacrifice the admiration of many men for the criticism of one, go ahead and get married.*
> Katherine Hepburn

If you are expecting too much – and no one is perfect – what happens when the initial rush of passion wears off and cracks appear? Do you try to fix them or just keep moving on to the next relationship and only staying around whilst it is still perfect? You may find that each relationship goes the same way after the initial passion fades.

But you could break this cycle. Be more tolerant of each other. Everyone is human. Try to understand your partner's way of thinking and try to keep the romance alive. Find time for each other and talk. Just because you have a partner doesn't mean that you have to live in each other's pockets.

> *When I'm alone, I can sleep crossways in bed without an argument.*
> Zsa Zsa Gabor

Keep some life of your own too. Every relationship needs to retain a little bit of mystery and a few harmless secrets.

> *I'm single for the first time in my life. I just want to be alone. I'm just going out with my sister and my girlfriends. It's cool not having to answer to anyone. I've never had time to get to know myself, I always put all of my energy into the man. I don't get to spend time on me. I'm just getting to know who I really am, until I can find someone else.*

Paris Hilton

> *When you're constantly looking for things from other people, you're not looking within yourself.*

Sandra Bernhard

> *I'm afraid of loneliness, but I don't see that being with someone is a safeguard against that.*

Baroness Susan Greenfield, scientist

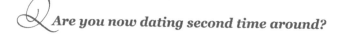 *Are you now dating second time around?*

A new relationship will make me feel better.

When you are looking for a new relationship, for that 'perfect' person to appear on the horizon, are you expecting this exciting new relationship to make you feel better about yourself?

A new relationship will not fix your problems. It may bring excitement and passion into your life, but it will not change how you feel about yourself and how you relate to others. To have a strong and well-balanced relationship with another person, you must love yourself first and then he/she will love you.

You cannot search for approval from another to endorse and uplift your own self-esteem.

It's also not necessary to give up yourself to love someone else. You have to love and respect yourself first and foremost before you can give to someone else.

You never know when you might meet someone. If you look, they don't come. New relationships happen in the most unexpected circumstances. Also, potential new lovers appear rather like buses. None at all or all at once.

> *I don't understand how a woman can leave the house without fixing herself up a little – if only out of politeness. And then, you never know, maybe that's the day she has a date with destiny. And it's best to be as pretty as possible for destiny.*
>
> Coco Chanel

You may find that once you are happily dating someone, others appear more interested too. Maybe when you are in demand you no longer look or appear as needy or possibly even desperate (even though you may have been unaware of this).

> *If only I knew then what I know now about boys and*
> *their mysterious ways, I would act just the same –*
> *loving them and hating them till the end of my days.*
>
> Helena Christensen

I am single and find the idea of dating again very scary.
It's all about being proactive, You are never going to meet someone by staying in watching the TV in your pyjamas. Cultivate your friendships with your single friends so you have someone to go out with. It's never too late to start afresh. There are many ways to start looking, from meeting friends of friends in your own circle to bars, singles events and online dating, which no longer has a social stigma.

I'm too old to start dating again.
You are never too old to start dating. You are as old as you feel. Look at Kim Cattrall, Teri Hatcher, Demi Moore, Sharon Stone. Yes, you say, they are all more successful, rich and beautiful. Of course they will have their own issues about getting older, but it's all about self-belief and confidence, whatever your age. I believe that there is someone for everyone, and that 'someone' appears when the time is right. As life moves on, so do your needs. But you need to feel good about yourself and happy with yourself before you find someone else you can be happy with.

> *Accept your age and the wisdom it brings.*
>
> Joan Collins

My next relationship will be my final serious, long term one leading to marriage.

Don't put so much pressure on yourself or your partner. Why don't you take this relationship day by day and see where it goes? You have much more chance of success and you won't frighten him off.

Why would anyone want me?

Because you're worth it. Just because someone else didn't want you, doesn't mean that no one else will. Be yourself. You will attract others by the signals you send out – positive body language together with how you dress and look. Acting or looking desperate, miserable or needy will not attract others – it will send them away.

> *There's no such thing as a plain woman. Everyone has attractive points so my advice is to accentuate your best assets.*
>
> Dita Von Teese

Do you always go for the wrong man?

I go for a man who is needy.

Don't make yourself feel wanted by trying to rescue or look after someone else, look after yourself first.

I go for the bad boys.

Ask yourself what you are gaining from these relationships. Do you live your life off an adrenalin rush and only want passion and excitement? Calm down and look at what you really want from a long term relationship.

> *I stayed in relationships that weren't right too long. I've since understood that, but I'm still very loyal.*
> Linda Evans

I choose boyfriends who bully me and treat me with disrespect and violence.

Don't feel that you are worthless and that it must be you that is causing them to act like this. Stop taking the blame. Don't keep forgiving them. Move on and find someone who treats you like a queen. You are worth it.

Do you think you could feel sexy again?

> *Being a sex symbol has to do with attitude, not looks. Most men think it's looks, most women know otherwise.*
> Kathleen Turner

What makes you feel sexy? Is it something you wear, (clothes or perfume), or something that someone says or does? Or have you forgotten what feeling sexy is? Feeling sexy is a state of mind and once you feel sexy you will look sexy.

It's about feeling self-confident and knowing that you look your best. If you feel gorgeous then that's how you'll look. If you feel good on the inside you will look good on the outside. Feeling sexy gives you a different walk, stance and attitude.

Learn to trust your mirror. Don't rely on others to tell you how you look and for compliments and endorsements. Accept what you see in the mirror and appreciate yourself. When you like your hair tell yourself how great it is, or that you look sexy in a dress. Don't be negative and see a couple of extra pounds you think you may have put on over the last few days. Re-affirm the positive.

How can you enhance your sex appeal?

I am not sure that I have any.

Everyone has sex appeal, but some have more of it than others and some know how to work it. Sex appeal doesn't disappear as you get older. In fact, it can become stronger with maturity and self-confidence. Sex appeal is not about what you are wearing, or even *not* wearing.

> *Men's traditional view of sexiness isn't sexy – it shouldn't be so obvious. Push-up bras and miniskirts? Sexiness to me is when people are comfortable with themselves.*
>
> Sienna Miller

It's about what you give off. But you have to feel confident in yourself to feel sexy. This is why we all love the naughty men who have a twinkle in the eye. They exude confidence and give off the message that they can have anyone they want.

Q Have you met your new man and are at the beginning stages of your relationship but want to make sure you don't make the same mistakes as you have done before?

I don't know whether to tell him the truth or play games.
There is no beating about the bush with later love as the need to appear cool seems to disappear when you reach your 40s and beyond. Also, there isn't a minute to waste! Life isn't a rehearsal. Directness can only be a better base from which to start a relationship as you know where you stand.

A man will never be able to read your mind. Don't play games. Be honest with each other. But maybe don't put all your cards on the table straight away and possibly be busy (or pretend to be) at least one night of the week!

I may be frightening him off.
Do you wait for him to call you or are you texting him before you even get home after the initial meeting? Are you so predatory that you are frightening him off? However much you may be lusting after a man, let him pursue you and feel like the hunter, not the prey.

> *A bit of lusting after someone*
> *does wonders for the skin.*
>
> Liz Hurley

Tips for making a relationship work

- Try always being affectionate and don't be afraid to show affection or kiss or hold his hands unexpectedly.
- Make sure you always communicate.
- Say what you really feel and don't hide your feelings.
- Be true to yourself and to him.
- Be honest.
- Listen to what he has to say.
- Understand him.
- Laugh together.
- Be kind.
- No one is perfect. Don't expect him to be.

> *I'm the kind of person who couldn't care less about sex*
> *until I meet someone who I think is wonderful. I sort of*
> *feel sorry for the next man who gets me. I may just have*
> *to kill him with passion.*
>
> Kirstie Alley

Q So, are you ready for sex with a new partner?

> *I married the first man I ever kissed. When I tell my children that they just about throw up.*
>
> Barbara Bush

How long should I wait before I have sex with my new man? How many dates?

> *The longer you wait before you have sex the better. As my grandmother used to say: why buy the whole cake if you can get a slice free?*
>
> Joan Collins

There is no exact answer to this; I have asked so many of my male friends their views.

There is the 'first date' theory: men don't marry girls who sleep with them on the first date. Then there is the 'third date' theory: three dates are enough time to get to know each other; enough to know that you want to take the relationship that stage further. Also that you aren't just dragging it out and wasting his time, or yours (even if the dinners were nice), as neither of you was just looking for another 'friend'.

It's often the men nowadays who wish to wait longer than you to commit to sex. Roles have reversed.

There is also the argument that if something feels right for both of you – why not?

But sex on a whim can lead to feelings of love for a person who is entirely wrong for you. Are you repeating a pattern of attraction to the wrong men?

I feel strange having a new boyfriend to stay in my home with my children.

This is a dilemma that happens to all single mothers at some time. If your children are small I would suggest that that no one stays over and meets them in the morning until you really know that this boyfriend is going to become a serious fixture in your life. If your children are old enough to have had their own adult relationships and understand, then it is really important to discuss how you all feel about a new man sleeping for the first time in your bed after their dad, and how they feel about it too.

Communication is all. You may find that they only want you to be happy, rather than be shocked that you now have a new partner and therefore a sex life.

The thought of sex with anyone new after all these years fills me with horror.

A good relationship, both in your everyday life and in the bedroom, is all about communication. Communicate your fears and thoughts and if your new partner loves you, he will listen to you and be understanding.

> *Sex is God's joke on human beings.*
>
> Bette Davis

I'm worried about someone new seeing me naked.

Childbirth and weight gain and loss, together with time and gravity, may have taken a toll on your body, but your new partner should be wanting you and loving you for the whole of who you are, not being super critical about you. If he is likely to be that critical then he is not the one for you.

If you happen to be dallying with a much younger man, he will have been attracted to you by your self-assurance, knowledge and sexual confidence that come with age and maturity, rather than your perfect body. If he just wanted that, he could date someone his own age.

As you should now be in the 'new you' frame of mind, you should have started to tone up your body with a healthy diet and exercise and feel good about yourself or, at least, be feeling more confident. You can always conceal and disguise those bits that you really can't change with soft lighting and well-fitting, sexy underwear. You'd be surprised at what men do and don't notice.

The best lovers do not necessarily have the best bodies. Your partner is not in bed with your cellulite or your stretch marks, he is in bed with you. Being comfortable and confident in your own skin, being able to laugh and be loving and giving will be far more appealing than a perfect body. Let your partner know whatever he is doing makes you feel wonderful and everything else will be forgotten.

> *My husband makes me feel very loved which gives me confidence. I know that affects how I look.*
>
> Liv Tyler

> *It's true that sex gets better with age. You stop comparing yourself to other people. You just have to relax and be yourself.*
>
> Janet Ellis

How will I know what to do after all these years of abstinence?
You will know. It's like riding a bicycle. You never forget...

> *Personally I know nothing about sex because I've always been married.*
>
> Zsa Zsa Gabor

> *You can love more than one person in your life, but things will be different. There'll be a different dynamic. Needs and desires change.*
>
> Francesca Annis

My last partner told me that I was no good in bed.
When you sleep with your new partner, it's very likely that you are about to find out that it was your last partner who was no good. Not *you* at all.

> *No surprise that women spend more time than men thinking about sex. There's rarely a moment I don't think about it. I have loads of sex in my head. The only difference between men and us is that we just don't have the time to do it.*
>
> Ulrika Johnston

I love my partner but it's not just about sex to me.
Everyone requires something different from their relationships. Some people need passion, others hot sex. But the best and longest lasting relationships work because you are both each other's best friend. But don't let all the hugs and kisses stop, as all human beings need some physical contact.

> *You know you truly have intimacy when you can totally be yourself.*
>
> Joan Collins

Tips to remember for the 'new you'

> *I always wanted to be somebody, but now I realize I should have been more specific.*
>
> Lily Tomlin

- Focus on one thing at a time. Then you won't feel dragged in too many directions.
- Make a small list of 'to do' tasks for each day. Not too

large. The list needs to be manageable. Tick them off as you do them and feel success when you look at the ticks at the end of the day.

- Don't feel guilty saying no. You don't have to please everybody all the time.
- Don't waste time getting wound up about small things. Put things into perspective.
- Allow others to help you, even if you don't think they'll do it as well as you.
- Make time for you.
- Drop 'if' and 'tomorrow' from your vocabulary.
- Stop criticising yourself.
- Stop judging yourself.
- Stop worrying what others think.
- Say sorry if you're wrong.
- Smile.

A small change can do a lot... And when you find things improving for you, accept and embrace them and be happy.

Now that we have taken this journey together, I hope that you are on the road to being that 'new you' you never imagined you could be.

Never forget that you are unique, have special qualities and always have something interesting to contribute to and bring to a partnership, friendship or a social occasion. Don't be too harsh on yourself, undervalue yourself or put yourself down.

You deserve to treat yourself and be treated as someone special.

Even if it takes you another year or even two to achieve your final destination of weight loss, learning a new skill to start a new career, or just making some new friends, you are now on the right road.

You now know all the ways to make yourself look and feel your best even if you don't implement them all at once. It's always about one step at a time. A little baby step, not a big leap.

Every so often you will come across an obstacle, a 'red traffic light' or even a diversion which will hold up your progress, but these things happen. Everyone is human It doesn't mean that you have to give up. Just pick yourself up and start again. Always look forward, never backward.

> *A woman is like a tea bag. It's only when she's in hot water that you realise how strong she is.*
> Nancy Reagan

> *Accept your age and the wisdom it brings.*
> Joan Collins

Accept yourself for you who are now, not who you were.

Allow yourself to change as you continue with your journey. Your view of the world and how the world views you will evolve along the way.

We are all on a continuous journey, just at different stages of it. Discovering your best you is all about you being the master of your own destiny. Don't leave it up to others. Create your own destiny.

Good luck on the rest of your journey.

Ceril's website

www.cerilcampbell.com

twitter: @cerilcampbell

Facebook: Ceril Campbell's Style Your Life